"This is a guidebook on how to rethink the way teachers teach, researchers think, and citizens make change. Building on a wide range of great thinkers—Thomas Kuhn on scientific creativity, Paulo Freire on learner-centered education, John Dewey on learning—Bilorusky lays out the steps through which we can do transformative action research. Based on his experience co-founding and heading the Western Institute for Social Research, he unites what we imagine as necessarily separate—the project of developing new ideas, mastering a discipline, working in community, building on diversity and making change. A highly important book on how to reshape our institutions and move forward in better ways."

— Arlie Hochschild, Professor Emerita of Sociology, University of California, Berkeley, author of *Strangers in Their Own Land: Anger and Mourning on the American Right*, a finalist for the National Book Award in 2016

"At last, we have an authoritative publication that details the foundation, methods, and important considerations of the 'the WISR way'—five decades of teaching, learning and doing Transformative Action Research at the Western Institute for Social Research. In Volume I, Dr. John Bilorusky and his colleagues offer a road map for researchers interested in a form of collaborative inquiry that encourages reflexivity and engagement as integral priorities, not options, for transformative social change. Hurrah!"

— Joyce. E. King, Benjamin E. Mays Endowed Chair for Urban Teaching, Learning & Leadership, College of Education & Human Development, Georgia State University, Past-President, The American Educational Research Association

"Berkeley's Western Institute for Social Research has been a premier undergraduate and graduate school for integrating multicultural academics and community-centered change. For fifty years teachers and students at this school have complemented the work of Ibram X. Kendi, bell hooks, Audre Lorde, Paulo Freire, and Myles Horton to promote community-based multicultural learning. This excellent volume examines approaches to conceptual and theoretical inquiry and shows how the school's activist scholars apply grounded theory, ethnography, authentic writing, and social transformation in the United States and around the world."

— T. D. Dickinson, Professor Emerita, Gender, Women and Sexuality Studies, Kansas State University

PRINCIPLES AND METHODS OF TRANSFORMATIVE ACTION RESEARCH

Principles and Methods of Transformative Action Research delves into both general principles and specific methods for basic steps in the action research process—asking questions, gathering and analyzing data, communicating findings, and pursuing action.

The role of collaboration is emphasized, with strategies of value to experts and engaged citizens in doing participatory research and community-based knowledge-building. Detailed attention is given to specific strategies of interviewing, participant observation, and judging and weighing evidence. The book draws on creative and critically minded elements of scientific traditions, such as transparency in telling the "story" of one's inquiry, identifying data that are "exceptions to the rule," and the value of non-formulaic, improvisational designs. Quite distinctively, the book addresses how to write in one's own voice, how to integrate action-and-inquiry into one's everyday life, issues of ethics and social responsibility, and how to consider both immediate, practical needs and "bigger picture," systemic challenges.

This book can serve as an undergraduate or graduate social sciences text on research methods. It is also a guidebook for action-oriented research by academics, professionals, and lay people alike, in community agencies, schools, and grassroots organizations, and for socially relevant academic research concerned with social justice, multiculturalism, and inclusiveness.

John A. Bilorusky (PhD, University of California, Berkeley) is co-founder of the Western Institute for Social Research in Berkeley. For 45 years, as a faculty member there, he has guided hundreds of student action research theses, dissertations, and projects, and consulted with dozens of community agencies and colleges on action research.

PRINCIPLES AND METHODS OF TRANSFORMATIVE ACTION RESEARCH

A Half Century of Living and Doing Collaborative Inquiry

John A. Bilorusky

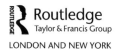

LONDON AND NEW YORK

First published 2021
by Routledge
2 Park Square, Milton Park, Abingdon, Oxon OX14 4RN

and by Routledge
52 Vanderbilt Avenue, New York, NY 10017

Routledge is an imprint of the Taylor & Francis Group, an informa business

© 2021 John A. Bilorusky

The right of John A. Bilorusky to be identified as author of this work has been asserted by him in accordance with sections 77 and 78 of the Copyright, Designs and Patents Act 1988.

All rights reserved. No part of this book may be reprinted or reproduced or utilised in any form or by any electronic, mechanical, or other means, now known or hereafter invented, including photocopying and recording, or in any information storage or retrieval system, without permission in writing from the publishers.

Trademark notice: Product or corporate names may be trademarks or registered trademarks, and are used only for identification and explanation without intent to infringe.

British Library Cataloguing-in-Publication Data
A catalogue record for this book is available from the British Library

Library of Congress Cataloging-in-Publication Data
Names: Bilorusky, John A. (John Alan), author.
Title: Principles and methods of transformative action research : a half century of living and doing collaborative inquiry / John A. Bilorusky.
Description: Abingdon, Oxon ; New York, NY : Routledge, 2021. | Includes bibliographical references and index. |
Identifiers: LCCN 2020047721 (print) | LCCN 2020047722 (ebook) | ISBN 9780367742423 (hardback) | ISBN 9780367742430 (paperback) | ISBN 9781003156741 (ebook)
Subjects: LCSH: Action research--Methodology. | Evaluation research (Social action programs)--Methodology.
Classification: LCC H62 .B523 2021 (print) | LCC H62 (ebook) | DDC 001.4--dc23
LC record available at https://lccn.loc.gov/2020047721
LC ebook record available at https://lccn.loc.gov/2020047722

ISBN: 978-0-367-74242-3 (hbk)
ISBN: 978-0-367-74243-0 (pbk)
ISBN: 978-1-003-15674-1 (ebk)

Typeset in Bembo
by Taylor & Francis Books

To those, no matter how oppressed or privileged,
who listen eloquently and who are motivated
by love, and by the pursuit of justice and collective well-being.

CONTENTS

List of illustrations   xiii
Acknowledgements   xiv
About the author   xvi
Contributing colleagues   xviii

PART I
The foundations   **1**

1 Introduction   5

   About me and my colleagues 5
   Aims of this book 7
   For whom is this book written, and why 9
   The Western Institute for Social Research—An "experimenting learning community" 10
   Trying to paint a nuanced picture of transformative action research 13

2 Principles, themes, and concepts   16

   All of us can create knowledge 16
   Some themes throughout the book 17
   What's involved in trying to be "transformative" 19

3 Building on intellectual traditions 22

   Thomas Kuhn, the structure of scientific revolutions: "Thinking outside the box" 22
   Qualitative, naturalistic methods and symbolic interactionism 27
   Transformative action-and-inquiry as transformative learning—Freire and Dewey 33
   Script-improvisation 34
   Developmental theories for transformative learning—Loevinger, the Dreyfus brothers, and Vygotsky 36
   Emotions matter in research 44
   The value and limitations of intellectual foundations—culture, gender, generation, and privilege in transformative action-and-inquiry 46

4 Research and society are interconnected 49

   Research as a social process 50
   Historical developments in social research and its underpinnings 58
   Concluding remarks 62

PART II
Methods of action research—steps in the process 63

5 Asking questions 65

   The importance of asking questions 65
   Asking questions about your community organization 68

6 Data-gathering and sampling 72

   Where do ideas and facts come from? 73
   Making it more conscious 77
   Sampling 81
   Broadening our experiences and information 83
   Note-taking to keep track of everyday observations and insights 90
   Interviewing strategies, issues, and considerations 92
   Eliciting ideas and information from others 101
   Analytical uses of group discussion 102

Contents **xi**

7 Data Analysis   105

*Seeking validity through transparency about one's research methods—
the alternatives to "bias" vs. "objectivity" 106
Making sense out of experiences 109
Judging the evidence 115
The dialectic of thought and action 125*

8 Communicating and collaborating   128

*The role of collaboration in action research and inquiry 128
Inquiry and others, learning from and with others—
"collaboration" 130
Communicating what we know to others 134
Putting ourselves at the heart of telling the story of our action-inquiry,
in our own voice 140
Writing in your own voice 144*

9 Issues and strategies of quantitative analysis   151

*Introduction 151
Demystifying statistics and quantitative vs. qualitative approaches to
weighing evidence 152
Rather than "hard" vs. "soft" data, consider different ways of thinking
about the world 161
Using graphs to think about data 163
The uses, misuses, and abuses of statistics 170*

PART III
**Important considerations in doing transformative
action research**   **175**

10 Immediate tasks and bigger picture   179

*Introductory considerations 179
Strains between "everyday life" and larger contexts 181
Looking for needed changes in the larger society and at underlying
systemic issues 182*

11 Inquiring more deeply   187

*Probing beneath the surface in our everyday lives in organizations and
communities 187*

12 Community knowledge-building   193

   *Stories, tangible details and "sensitizing concepts," especially in
      participatory research 194*
   Good science, making it public and valid 195
   Qualities of knowledge-building 196

13 Ethical considerations   198

   Ethical issues in protecting research participants 199
   *Ethical issues in formulating the purposes and design of an action
      research project 201*
   "Social responsibility" and transformative action research 201

14 Concluding remarks   205

   *More for the interested reader—brief highlights of what will be addressed
      in Volume 2—Action research: Uses and illustrations of
      transformative inquiry 210*

References   212
Index   216

ILLUSTRATIONS

Figures

9.1 Four graphs showing the percent of people in each of four hypothetical groups consuming different amounts of sugary beverages each week   156
9.2 The shapes of three different normal distributions   163
9.3 The shapes of two different bi-modal distributions   165
9.4 Five graphs showing significantly different relationships between two variables: Three exponential and two linear   167
9.5 Two graphs depicting chaos and discontinuity   168
9.6 A scatterplot graph approximating a linear relationship   170

Table

3.1 Parallels between Dreyfus Theory of Stages of Expert Knowledge, Loevinger's Stages of Ego Development and Four Curricular Models   39

Box

Steps in the process of action research   63

ACKNOWLEDGEMENTS

As the subtitle of this book suggests, this book, and its companion book, *Cases and Illustrations of Transformative Action Research: Five Decades of Collaborative Action and Learning,* are literally the results of over 50 years of learning, inquiry, practice and collaboration. I wish to acknowledge especially my colleagues of many years, the late Terry F. Lunsford and Cynthia Lawrence, who contributed so much to the process of developing transformative action research, and consequently, to this book.

I thank Torry Dickinson and Brian Gerrard for encouraging me to write these two books. Torry has done so for many years, and Brian, gave me the last needed impetus, along with the "extra time" due to having to shelter in place during Covid-19. Brian has read and commented on a number of drafts of portions of both books, and Torry has made valuable suggestions about important points and ideas to include.

The importance and value of collaboration, of learning from and with others cannot be emphasized enough. I cannot possibly list all the many people who contributed to my understanding and use of transformative action research. Many key people have been acknowledged throughout the book. Because my understanding of action research has developed especially since 1975 hand in hand in the experimenting multicultural learning community that is the Western Institute for Social Research (WISR), here, I wish to acknowledge many, but my no means all, of the people who have been crucial contributors to this rather distinctive academic institution that many of affectionately refer to as "wiser." Listed in alphabetical order are just some of the amazing students and alumni, faculty, Board and friends of WISR with whom have I had the good fortune to collaborate: Victor Acosta, Fernando Alegria*, Richard Allen, Peggy Baxter, John Bear, Larry Berkelhammer, Robert Blackburn*, J. Herman Blake, Uwe Blesching, John Borst, Janet McAfee Bowman, Marcia Campos, Che Kum Clement, Margery Coffey, Torry Dickinson, Rich Douglas, Sevgi Fernandez, Makhosazana Fletcher, Steven Fletcher, Brian Gerrard, Chuck Greene, Linda

Acknowledgements xv

Hartling, Dennis Hastings, Paul Heist*, Milly Henry, Gabriela Hofmeyer, Marilyn Jackson, Joanne Kowalski*, Vera Labat, Cynthia Lawrence, Richard Lawrence, J.C. (Calu) Lester*, Dalia Liang, Na Limopasmanee, Larry Loebig, Terry Lunsford*, Ronald Mah, Marilyn (Lindi) Martin, Roger Mason, Eric Mauer, Michael McAvoy*, Sudia Paloma McCaleb, Agnes Morton, Antonia Pantoja*, Wilhelmina Perry, Jacob Perea, Deborah Pruitt, Suzanne Quijano, Rosa Reinikainen, Mona Scott, Monika Scott, Shyaam Shabaka, Sajad Shakoor, Jake Sloan, Anngwyn St. Just, Mary Suzuki, Oba T'Shaka, Dorothy Terrell*, James Todd, III*, Andrea Turner, Barbara Valentino*, Karen Wall, Art Warmoth*, John Watkins, David Yamada (*deceased).

I wish to acknowledge and thank Hannah Shakespeare, of Routledge Press, for her strongly encouraging and extremely communicative support from the initial stages of reviewing this book, and forward to completion. There are many others at Routledge, not known to me by their names, working behind the scenes, who have made important and valued contributions.

Finally, the action-and-inquiry in which I have been engaged over the years, and indeed all my life's endeavors, have been nurtured and guided by the love I have so fortunately shared with my immediate family—with my late mother, Arzelia Bilorusky, my late, grandmother, Mattie Ann Butterfass, my wife of 25 years, Janet Staab Bilorusky, and my three adult children, Clark, Kyle, and Nicole. Further, I wish to acknowledge the special experience of sharing love and collaborating with my wife, Janet, in raising our twins, Kyle and Nicole over the past 22+ years.

ABOUT THE AUTHOR
John A. Bilorusky, PhD

John is President of Western Institute for Social Research (WISR), was a co-founder of WISR in 1975, and has served full-time on WISR's faculty ever since. During that time, he has supervised over 100 student dissertations, Master's theses, and undergraduate senior theses on a wide range of topics, almost all of which have used action research methods, and he has guided and mentored students in the conduct of hundreds of other action research projects. These projects have been conducted in a variety of settings, and by students with many different interests and levels of previous professional and community experience, from all walks of life, and from many varied cultural backgrounds.

After graduating with his Bachelor's degree from the University of Colorado with honors in physics and honors in general studies (1967), John changed fields of study earned his PhD in Higher Education at the University of California, Berkeley, in 1972.

In 1970–71, John taught senior thesis seminars in the Social Sciences Integrated Courses and Field Major, as a Teaching Associate at the University of California, Berkeley. From 1971 to 1973, he was Assistant Professor of Urban Affairs and Senior Research Associate in the Institute for Research and Training in Higher Education at the University of Cincinnati. There he taught the required action research course in the College of Community Services, created and coordinated the College's Individualized Learning Program, and served as an in-house organizational and evaluation consultant for faculty at the university. Then, from 1973 to 1975, he was Director of Graduate Studies at University Without Walls-Berkeley.

He is the author of published articles and papers on higher education and social change, adult learning, and practical community-based and participatory research methods, including a co-authored book published by the Carnegie Commission on Higher Education, *May 1970: The Campus Aftermath of Cambodia and Kent State* (with Richard Peterson). He has served as a consultant for community agencies in the area of participatory action research, including directing a major study of needs and services for low-income elders for the Los Angeles Community Redevelopment Agency, and using participatory research in collaboration with the Bay Area Black United Fund on three occasions for their African American Health Summits. In addition, he has done collaborative consultations with dozens of Bay Area groups over the years. He has conducted evaluations of colleges and educational innovations, for such institutions as De Pauw University (Indiana), Macalester College (Minnesota), Colorado College, New College of California, and Fresno State University. He has conducted feasibility studies for such groups as the California Housing Trust Fund and Cleveland State University's Department of Human Services.

He was Director of WISR's nationwide demonstration project, under a grant from the U.S. Department of Education's Fund for the Improvement of Postsecondary Education (FIPSE) from 1980 to 1983—on extending the teaching, learning, and use of action research throughout the larger community. John serves on the Advisory Board of the global network of Human Dignity and Humiliation Studies (https://www.humiliationstudies.org/).

CONTRIBUTING COLLEAGUES

The late Terry F. Lunsford, JD, PhD: Terry's academic career began with his earning a BA with honors in General Studies and Humanities from the University of Chicago (1951). He did pre-doctoral study in Psychology at the University of Chicago 1951–1954, and went on to get the JD in Law there (1957). After beginning his academic career, he received a PhD in Sociology at the University of California at Berkeley, in 1970. Terry taught at UC Berkeley for four years, where he also was Chair of the Social Sciences Integrated Courses & Field Major, Academic Director of the Field Studies Program, and a professional researcher at the Center for the Study of Higher Education, at the Health & Medical Sciences Program, and at the Institute for the Study of Social Change. He was involved in the early years of studying the social and legal impacts of genetic research. He used his expertise in law and his extensive experience in and knowledge of interviewing when he worked on the National Jury Project in Oakland, training lawyers in methods for interviewing prospective jurors. He served on the faculty and the Board of the WISR for over 30 years until his death.

Cynthia Lawrence, PhD: Cynthia was a schoolteacher for many years before becoming a faculty member in Teacher Education at the University of California, San Diego, with expertise in the areas of multicultural education, alternative education, and the teaching of language skills. She then earned her PhD in Higher Education and Social Change, from WISR, 1987, after which she became a member of WISR's faculty for 25 years and is currently core faculty emeritus at WISR and serves on WISR's Board. She is an expert in the areas of multicultural education, alternative education, and the teaching and learning of language skills. She is a retired faculty member in Teacher Education at the University of California, San Diego. Over the years, she has developed materials and conducted training sessions to heighten teachers' sensitivity to multicultural issues. She has conducted workshops on interracial issues for such groups as the Family Stress Center and the National Organization for Women (NOW). She was appointed in 1991 to the San Diego Human Relations Commission.

PART I
The foundations

This book is about "research," "inquiry," and "action," and an overall perspective on methods for bringing those together in transformative ways to make a difference. Most people use "action research" to describe and discuss research that is used in conjunction with action, whether before, during or after the action taking place. The word "transformative" in "transformative action research" means several things.

First, action and research, or action-and-inquiry, transform each other, where each action-and-inquiry is a different emphasis, but still part of a yin-yang sort of whole. Consider for example, "imaginative and reflective action" which refers to inquiring aspects of action, or "engaged and involved inquiry" which refers to the action-oriented qualities of research and inquiry.

Second, "transformative action research" leads to some changes that "matter," that are meaningful, valuable, and useful for an individual, a group, an organization, a community, and/or the larger society.

"Transformative" action research is not limited to cut-and-dried processes, but often uses improvised strategies, still based on solid principles of inquiry. Consequently, it may often lead to significant changes, for even if the changes are small, they may not merely be incremental ones along already well-known paths, but instead lead to fundamentally different directions and outcomes.

Further, *"action research methods" often refer to a constellation of procedures, and considerations, to conduct a careful and well-designed study or project, most often culminating in a written product as well as perhaps some action steps.* I've decided to use the terms "inquiry" and "action-and-inquiry" to refer to everyday activities, even if not part of a formally designed project. Any one of us can inquire into the meaning of something we notice or observe, read in the papers, or see on TV or the Internet. "Inquiry" often has the connotation of critical and/or imaginative thinking—not unlike Archimedes' unanticipated insight in his bathtub, whereupon he reportedly ran down the street naked shouting "Eureka!" That is an example of action-and-inquiry—the action of stepping into the water, with the observation of the level of the water rising and this resulting in his insight about the solution of the problem of how to measure the volume of an irregularly shaped object.

In this book, I often use the word "transformative" to emphasize that I am especially interested in how action research and action-inquiry can be used to bring about fundamentally new insights, practices, and change—not unlike Archimedes' everyday life breakthrough in solving a problem he had been pondering for some time. Each and every one of us can increase our likelihood of such "Eureka (I've found it!)" experiences by making a regular practice of trying to engage in transformative action-and-inquiry, whether in formal projects or as part of our everyday lives.

Action-and-inquiry during the Covid-19 pandemic

At the time, I'm writing this book, we're in the midst of the Covid-19 pandemic, and lots of ideas and information are swirling around regarding causes, and possible solutions, to an easily contagious virus that seems to act in ways that are very much outside the realm of what we experience with various strains of flu viruses. How do we "know" which information to pay the most attention to? What should we believe? Why? Experts say something one week, emphasizing that the main dangers are damage to our lungs, then a couple of weeks later, it seems a risk is blood clotting and even strokes. Maybe both are true—probably they are. How do we think about these unfolding "facts"—scientists and medical professionals themselves are challenged in their research laboratories, and those of us who are "lay people" have to decide which precautions to take—to protect ourselves, our loved ones, and strangers as well. These issues of "inquiry" have "action" implications, and inevitably we make decisions that are emotional—if I go outside to walk, or even jog, should I wear a face mask, or should I just keep my distance? Should we wait to go back to business as usual until there is a strongly proven treatment? And, if so, what does "strongly proven" mean? Should we wait until there is a proven vaccine? What's "strongly proven" to one person may be tenuous to another. How do we decide? Some believe there is nothing to really worry about unless you're over 60 or 70 or have a significant chronic health problem. Similarly, government leaders and policy makers must make decisions about what laws and guidelines to pass.

There are ethical dilemmas in many of our everyday actions, and right now, people are making decisions about how much to risk more deaths, as compared with increased unemployment, or alternatively, with a major decline in the stock market. For each of us, out of self-interests, concerns for our loved ones, or for the well-being of others in our community or the larger society, we have been thrown, out of necessity, into having to do action-and-inquiry. The alternatives are to go with our "gut instincts" or "personal beliefs and preferences" alone. To be sure, action research projects, and everyday action-and-inquiry, always also involve gut instincts, beliefs, and preferences, and of course our values and commitments. We needn't deny or "eliminate" our emotions, beliefs, and values, but try to harness them and keep them in perspective, by using principles and methods of action research and inquiry to guide and aid us in gaining insights and making decisions.

About the first four chapters

In the introductory three chapters, I share highlights about my own history, especially the history of my collaborations with others. *As I will emphasize throughout this book, collaboration is invaluable whether one is doing a formal action research project or engaged in everyday action-and-inquiry* (see especially Chapter 8). I discuss how and why I see this book to be of potential value to people from many walks of life from academia to grassroots activism, to citizen participation, to school and agency improvement efforts, among others. I highlight some intellectual traditions that have been of special value—scientific traditions, qualitative and naturalistic research and grounded theory, human development, theories of adult learning and social learning, and epistemology and expert knowledge.

Transformative action-and-inquiry is very much about "learning," and it works hand-in-glove with collaborative, improvisational, learner-centered education. Indeed, the tiny, very innovative degree-granting institution, the Western Institute for Social Research (https://www.wisr.edu) has been an "experimenting community" that has attracted many committed and inquisitive faculty and students over the years, and consequently, it has served as a collaborative, hospitable context for developing and refining methods of "transformative action research." Chapter 4 explores some of the significant ways in which research and society impact one another.

How to approach reading this book

First, the reader should keep in mind that my epistemological, theoretical framework on action research methods is not one that I will neatly package and articulate in any one place in this book, but rather it is to be discerned by reading through this book to gain a holistic sense of the situationally variable, nuanced ways in which I, and others, have pursued and used transformative action research. Second, although I've included examples of applications of action research throughout this book, the strongly interested reader will find that there are many more illuminating examples in the companion book, *Cases and Stories of Transformative Action Research: Five Decades of Collaborative Action and Learning* (Bilorusky, 2021). The general principles, and various methods of Transformative Action Research become increasingly meaningful and useful as one examines a greater number of specific examples.

1
INTRODUCTION

About me and my colleagues

In this book on the transformative power of some approaches to action research, I am drawing on over 50 years of learning—as a student, a faculty member, and a community-engaged and inquiring citizen. I have been involved as a faculty member at the Western Institute for Social Research (WISR—https://www.wisr.edu/welcome) since founding it with three others in 1975. During the past 45 years, I have learned from and with WISR students and faculty more than I can ever put into words, but I will try to articulate some important lessons from the myriad of ways we have used action research. Together, we have learned much about transformative inquiry as a way of living—through our actions, heartfelt commitments, intellectual curiosity, and dedication to learning for both personal and societal transformations.

Going back to the 1960s, I have benefited from learning from, and with, many inspiring, open-hearted, socially responsible, and intellectually engaged people. I could not possibly name all those with whom I have had the good fortune to collaborate, but I will single out several people. The late Dr. Walter Weir (head of the honors program at the University of Colorado throughout the 1960s) taught and demonstrated the joy of learning and that ideas can matter and make a difference in our lives. As a graduate student I benefited from encouragement from Dr. Paul Heist (Professor of Higher Education at UC Berkeley) and Dr. Arlie Hochschild (then, a young faculty member in Sociology at UC Berkeley), who encouraged me to find my own voice, in matters of educational and societal transformation.

Immediately after finishing graduate school, I took a faculty position at the University of Cincinnati. There, with my colleague, the late Dr. Harry Butler, we tried to put into practice some of the principles of action-and-inquiry for transformative learning, during our two years together as faculty at the University of Cincinnati. Harry went on to become Dean of Social Work, San Diego State University, 1975–78. He then left academia and spent three decades in private practice as Licensed Clinical Social Worker in San Diego. We continued to exchange ideas and give one another mutual support as friends for almost 50 years, until his recent passing in December 2019.

My good friend and colleague, first at UC Berkeley and then at WISR, the late, Dr. Terry F. Lunsford, was always ready to pose questions and to engage in dialogue with me about matters of learning, action-inquiry, and social change. Further, I learned, or at least tried to learn, from his knack for articulating complex ideas in down-to-earth ways, without academic jargon. Terry was a key faculty member at WISR in the 1980s and 1990s, and we worked together on WISR's U.S. Department of Education-funded nationwide demonstration project on how to extend the teaching and learning of action research methods throughout the larger community. Terry and I collaborated in writing curriculum materials for that project, many of which I have drawn on, by revising and updating them, in writing this book.

Terry brought to our collaboration expertise in law, organizational dynamics, and sociology. He had a JD from the University of Chicago and a PhD in Sociology from UC Berkeley. He was a skillful in understanding and communicating how to combine theory and practice in the social sciences. Terry taught at UC Berkeley for four years, where he also was Chair of the Social Sciences Integrated Courses and Field Major, and then became Academic Director of the Field Studies Program there. At Berkeley, he was also a professional researcher at the Center for the Study of Higher Education, at the Health and Medical Sciences Program, and at the Institute for the Study of Social Change. He was involved in the early years of studying the social and legal impacts of genetic research. He used his expertise in law and his extensive experience in and knowledge of interviewing when he worked on the National Jury Project in Oakland, training lawyers in methods for interviewing prospective jurors. Beyond the breadth and depth of his knowledge, Terry was always open to dialogue and collaboration. His sensibilities and nuanced understanding of the many uses of action research are in evidence throughout this book.

Quite especially, I have learned much about transformative action-and-inquiry, as an integral quality in the pursuit of social change, community improvements, learner-centered education, and inclusiveness, by continually discussing ideas and strategies for promoting transformative learning with my WISR colleague and friend of 40 years, Dr. Cynthia Lawrence. I had the good fortune to begin our collaboration while she was a doctoral student at WISR in the early1980s. At that time, she was also a full-time faculty member in Teacher Education at the University of California, San Diego, following her many years as a schoolteacher focusing on alternative education, multicultural education, and the development of language skills. Soon after completing her WISR PhD, she joined WISR's faculty for over

20 years until her retirement. Cynthia was also, like most students and faculty at WISR, very involved in her community. In San Diego, she conducted workshops on interracial issues, was one year's Grand Marshall for the Gay Freedom Day parade and served on the San Diego Human Relations Commission in the early 1990s.

Our collaboration was built on a valuable combination of having much in common (intangible ways of seeing the world and thinking about things), and by contrast, of having many life experiences that were quite different. White males, even those of us who are not particular affluent, have privileges that easily go unnoticed, and an extremely talented and well-educated African American woman, who identifies as lesbian, faces many layers of obstacles and challenges, not to mention everyday insults, that are not so easy for the rest of us to understand. Together, we forged a partnership in working with students, and in advancing WISR's distinctive learning methods (including the transformative action research methods). We valued those quite unusual moments when we would see things differently, for it was then that we knew that with further discussion we could gain deeper insights.

Other faculty and students at WISR have been invaluable colleagues as well, and there are literally dozens who have helped me to learn about action research and about living life engaged in action-and-inquiry, that is about learning. These friends, family, and colleagues have contributed to the meaning I have found in my work for a half century now, and beyond that to my life. My mother, Arzelia Bilorusky, who lived in every decade of the 20th century, gave me a foundation for transformative learning by modeling and teaching me the importance of caring for others, using conversation to think things through and to envision new possibilities, and to have an eagerness always to learn more.[1] Finally, and not at all insignificantly, my entire family—my three children, Clark, Kyle, Nicole, and my wife, Janet, have given me love, support, opportunities to learn and grow. One of the important messages of this book is that collaboration and learning with others is critical to transformative inquiry, as well as to a joyful and meaningful life!

Aims of this book

This book is designed to engage the reader in two ways to use "transformative action research" or as I sometimes refer to it, "transformative action-and inquiry":

- first, for "living life" and continually learning, especially in collaboration with others (i.e., pursuing transformative action-and-inquiry), and
- second, for "doing" a research project" or doing transformative action research.

So, *"transformative action-inquiry" may be seen as a way of living, and learning, of combining thinking and acting in one's life, in order to bring about personal and/or societal transformations.* Many things must go together—getting information, having rich experiences, or making observations must go along with critical reflection, collaboration, and dialogue with others. To this we must add imaginatively asking new questions and making concerted efforts to try out in action our emerging insights. Much more can be extremely valuable—looking at both the immediate tasks and the bigger picture, probing beneath the surface of first appearances, participating in one's community or group, identifying and sharing insightful stories and illustrative experiences, and engaging in improvisations from one's initially scripted methods, and using paradigms as springboards for transformative efforts, rather than being bound by them. I will discuss these qualities in greater depth and detail throughout the book.

Further, *I hope that this book will provide valuable guidance for those who want to "do" action research.* We will consider different "steps" of action research methodology. Although these "stages" or steps are analytically useful, they do *not* necessarily need to be done in the neat sequence outlined here, and in the precise sequence that some texts present as the "right" way to do action research. We will almost always need to improvise, to revise our next steps, based on what we are learning during the process of inquiry. To help us focus on key domains of action research, it is nonetheless useful to note the following stages or steps, each of which is addressed in detail in Part II:

1. defining the problem(s) and asking questions;
2. identifying what data (information/experience) are relevant, given the problem identified, the questions asked, and/or the purposes and commitments that are guiding our actions and/or research;
3. identifying the "best" or "most feasible" sources of data, ideally trying to "sample for diversity" and inclusiveness, including looking for exceptions to the rule and/or unusual, but relevant circumstances;
4. "gathering" the data (making observations, interviewing others, or surveying people, for example);
5. making "sense" of the data—analyzing and critically reflecting on the data, comparing "slices" of data, weighing evidence that may point in varied directions, and synthesizing data and looking for themes/patterns, including identifying variations or exceptions to the themes, and "grounding" or illustrating the themes (generalizations and concepts) and variations with a variety of apt, relevant examples or stories;
6. formulating and communicating to others, the "findings—what we think we know," "for now," and then making some recommendations for action/ practice, and identifying questions for further study and research; and
7. taking some action or doing some further research and jumping back into any of the above domains or steps—and continuing the process.

In many formally designed research studies, or action research projects, these stages are often seen as sequential; yet, in actual practice, it is usually productive, to recycle through one item more than one time before getting to the later items. Sometimes, "two" items happen together—in gathering data, we may unavoidably notice ("analyze") something which leads a new question (item #1) which in turn motivates us to think about further, new efforts to look for different data, or new sources of data, and so on.

For whom is this book written, and why

This book is especially for people who aim to change for the better, their communities, organizations, educational institutions, and the society. Why? First, *I believe that in a democratic society where we can together pursue such important ideals as social and racial justice, equality and environmental sustainability, the more of us who are engaged in collaborating, the better. Better still if we join in action-and-inquiry with people from all walks of life.*

Why else? *I have had the good fortune to collaborate and make use of action research, both through formally designed projects, as well as in informal and continuing action-and-inquiry, with people from the following groups*:

- innovative professional researchers and consultants concerned with matters of community participation, social change and justice, and diversity and inclusiveness;
- people working in community service agencies, whether in positions of authority and/or on the "front lines";
- grassroots and neighborhood activists, and concerned citizens;
- intellectual activists and independent scholars concerned with both specific topics and broad issues of fundamental social change, laws, and policies;
- classroom teachers who wish to engage their students in action research, or even possibly include other teachers or parents in the process;
- innovatively-minded college professors teaching research courses, especially those with a "hand-on" learner-centered approach, and who wish to inspire and guide their students into meaningful research activities, and still covering much of the standard research methods content found in required course, but in fairly down-to-earth language;
- students and scholars interested in broadening their understanding of the many ways in which qualitative research methods can be used in action research;
- innovatively-minded liberal arts professors, who may find much of value here—about critical reflection, imaginative inquisitiveness, self-directed learning and writing in one's own voice—things that address many of the traditional high ideals and missions of liberal education; and quite broadly and especially
- people who wish to develop methods of inquiry, which consider and make use of, the insights of varied perspectives—including multi-generational, cultural, and gender, and importantly also issues of privilege and marginalization.

Indeed, people from all walks of life and domains of experience might join together to form action research teams and cooperate with each other actively, and get the benefit of the insights that are so often monopolized, today, by the big research institutions and their specialized experts. The kinds of action research discussed in this book are designed so that they can also be done by non-professional researchers, who are engaged in doing rather than only studying, and who want to use their research for the improvement of their communities.

Gaps addressed by this book

In writing this book, I've tried to include ideas, perspectives and specific illustrations that will help to fill in what I see to be gaps in many other books.

- Many books on action research are written as guides for dissertations or theses, or as textbooks to introduce students to a comprehensive set of procedures deemed essential to creating a valid and systematically designed research project. These books leave unaddressed a whole host of situational complexities which are often encountered when one wants to make use of action research in a "real world" application, or when we wish to integrate action-and-inquiry into our everyday lives, not as finite, time-limited projects, but to continue to learn and to try to make a difference in the world.
- Unlike this book, more practically oriented books focus only on one setting, for example on teachers working with students, or organizational consultants working to serve the goals of those in positions of authority who pay for their services. Certainly, the interests of workers in organizations is not at all always the same as the interests of the people with the authority and resources to hire an action research consultant.
- Many books on research look at things mostly from the point of view of the "person" who is "the researcher." Here, I have written this book with the intention that those "conducting" action research should aim to broaden participation to include those who are sometimes excluded, and to collaborate, to the extent possible, with people in a variety of roles impacted by the action research. For this reason, many people value "*participatory* action research."

The Western Institute for Social Research—An "experimenting learning community"

An academic institution and an experimenting learning community

With three others I founded WISR in 1975 as a tiny, nonprofit, experimental academic degree-granting institution. Since then, we have offered California licensed degrees—Bachelor's, Master's and Doctoral degrees in several related, interdisciplinary areas: community leadership and justice, education and community leadership, marriage and family therapy (counseling psychology), and education and social change. Our mission has been to emphasize personalized learner-centered education, with emphases on action research, inclusiveness in a multicultural learning community, and an inquiring commitment to the pursuit of social justice and change. And do so, keeping costs low and tuition affordable (currently $7,500/year). As noted earlier, our distinctive mission has attracted a remarkable and diverse group of faculty and students—people interested in inquiry and in action, and people who have been motivated to try to make constructive contributions to others and the society as a whole (Bilorusky & Lawrence, 2003). *We sometimes refer to ourselves as an "experimenting learning community" because part of our mission is for WISR to be a welcoming and inclusive space in which people can come together, to collaborate and be intentional "experimenting" in trying to come up with creative ideas and practices, to improve professions, communities, and even the larger society.*

WISR's learners

Our students, ages 21 to 80, and with many varied identities, have come primarily from these groups:

- community service professionals, especially those who are progressive and concerned with multiculturality and social justice, and who want to create reforms and even major changes within their agencies, communities, or professions;
- community activists, usually with progressive agendas concerned with the needs and purposes of the marginalized groups with whom they are working, or with bringing about larger social policy and/or education for social change goals;
- college professors and other educators, including adult and community educators, who share some of the progressive and social change agendas noted above; and
- therapists who wish to pursue advanced studies in innovative areas within their profession, such as trauma therapy, somatic therapy, and therapeutic approaches that also concern social change.

Action research and learner-centered collaboration

In our one-on-one mentoring and collaboration with students, and in small group seminars we have encouraged students to do action research projects on topics of strong personal interest throughout their studies at WISR, and especially in their culminating thesis or dissertation. Transformative action research, or action-and-inquiry, is fundamentally about learning. Further, my decades of experience have convinced me that, overall, learner-centered approaches to learning are most effective, especially because learners make use of what they have learned in ways that are significant and meaningful to them. In important respects, this book is about "learning." Indeed, action research, and the synthesis of "action" and "inquiry," the yin and the yang of a meaningful whole, are about learning, about personal transformation, and the transformation of the groups, organizations, and society in which we live. In many ways, this book is about "learning how to learn."

In part, this book can be an aid to a collaborative, and sometimes also a mentoring, process. The process must begin with the learner and their interests, their passions, and the questions and purposes that are important to them. If the learner's questions change, or their interests, and purposes evolve, then so must the direction of the action-and-inquiry, or the action research project. The learner's voice—anyone "using action research" is a learner—must be at the center of the process. Ideally, the learner will find others with whom to collaborate. It's ok that some efforts may be mostly solitary. When there are opportunities for collaboration with others who are at least "mostly compatible" in terms of values and interests, then so much the better. Efforts aimed at community or organizational transformation are greatly aided by broad-based collaboration and participation.

In 1980, WISR received a major, three-year grant from the U.S. Department of Education's Fund for the Improvement of Postsecondary Education (FIPSE)—to serve as a nationwide demonstration project on teaching, learning, and using action research throughout the larger community. Our FIPSE-funded project from 1980 to 1983 focused on community agency staff but included activists and educators as well.

During that project, WISR faculty, especially Terry Lunsford and myself, developed curriculum materials and articles. At first, for over a year, and on a weekly basis, Terry and I would together discuss what topics we wanted to write about, and then spend an hour or two beginning to discuss that topic. At some point, Terry would often interview me about my further ideas about that topic, or method. Then, he would draft something based on a combination of both of our thoughts. Then, I would take that draft and make revisions. We might work on the resulting draft further. Other times, I would draft something for Terry to read and comment on, and we would discuss, and make further revisions. Beyond the initial three years in the early 1980s, we spent many hours over more than a couple of years in his living room working on these things together, and doing so at a time when we would draft things partly in handwriting, and partly using a computer, or even a typewriter!

Further, for many years after this project, I collaborated extensively with Dr. Cynthia Lawrence and Dr. Terry Lunsford, as well as others at WISR, including especially, Vera Labat, MPH—to develop added writings, and important insights, all of which I've now revised, updated, and published for the first time in this book. I know from years of personal experience how important collaboration is to transformative action research.

More and more, we talked about the importance of these kinds of methods of inquiry in supporting the efforts of people to engage in "community-based knowledge-building." Similar to the community development activists from around the world who have promoted "participatory research," we have always believed in the innate potential of everyone to create important knowledge from their own experiences, which in turn will contribute to the knowledge, actions, and experience of others.

A key emphasis of our approach to inquiry has been to help people to become more aware of methods they can use, within the context of their everyday experiences and lives that support their roles as builders of knowledge. We want people to be aware that they *already are* builders of knowledge, even if they don't consciously realize it. To this end, qualitative research methods like participant observation and interviewing are valuable tools, as will be discussed in great detail in Chapter 6.

How can observations go deeper beneath the surface? How can we critique and refine the validity of the insights from our observations and experiences? How can we more pointedly and astutely learn from our conversations with others? Are there people with whom we should talk (or "interview" if you like) who will provide important insights to which we don't yet have enough awareness or access? Are there some things that we can read that will provide alternative perspectives or fresh ("out of the box") frameworks for reflecting on and analyzing our insights and experiences? How can we learn to look at the "bigger picture" while maintaining an appropriate concern with the pressing "immediate tasks" that require our attention? These are the kinds of issues that we explore, and we use tools from qualitative research, the discovery of grounded theory, participatory research, even cutting-edge knowledge-building in the natural sciences, among other paradigms to help ourselves and our learners to fashion tools and perspectives to further enhance our action-oriented inquiries. These and other traditions of importance to transformative action-and-inquiry, to "action research, the WISR Way" will be considered in some depth in Chapter 3.

Trying to paint a nuanced picture of transformative action research

Over the years, many people have asked me why we use the term "action research" to characterize our methods on learning, inquiry, and action at WISR. I tell them, quite candidly, that this term may be misleading, since it grew out of early efforts in the mid-1970s, at a time when we were mostly concerned with distinguishing WISR's approach to research from aloof, traditional academic approaches that were often unconcerned with "action." As will be discussed in Chapter 3, our methods have drawn on several traditions, including "qualitative research" in the social sciences, the "best" of mainstream scientific methods, and "participatory research" promoted by some community and international activists. Building on such traditions, and based on our own evolving endeavors, faculty, students, and alumni of WISR have developed, refined, and articulated methods which put forth some specific nuances and emphases that we have come to appreciate.

To better understand WISR's notions of "action research" in a larger context, it may be helpful to mention briefly a few "types" of research practiced by others. These include:

- Experimental design which comes out of the logical positivist, behaviorist traditions, and especially psychology where that field has often been "competing" with hard sciences for credibility. Experimental design attempts to "control" variables in specially constructed research settings (sometimes "labs") where "subjects" are often randomly assigned to either a "control" or "experimental" group. Unlike our approach to action research, these studies are done in a special setting that is *not* part of everyday, naturally occurring social realities.
- Survey research focuses on the counting frequency of occurrences in specific populations, such as in surveying public opinion on various current issues of the day.

- Qualitative research is meaning-focused inquiry, growing out of symbolic interactionism, and is one of a few, major schools of thought in sociology. I, and others, at WISR have been greatly influenced by this tradition.
- "Action research"—outside of WISR, and prior to 1970—was oftentimes the concern of professionals in such applied fields as business and organizational development, especially to have practical applications within mainstream organizations.
- "Participatory research" gained interest among activists internationally in the 1970s, and was often part of a community development-oriented movement concerned with mobilizing masses of (usually oppressed) people to engage in inquiry that could help them to transform the circumstances of their lives.

In discussing the development of transformative action research at WISR, I am not able to present one formula, or precisely defined approach, but rather will try to paint a realistic, and nuanced, picture of different ways that action research can be done. My aims in this book are to show how:

- "Research" can take many forms, including but not limited to, formally designed projects that are systematic, and that use carefully crafted procedures of data collection and analysis, culminating in a written product.
- "Research" can be seen as "everyday inquiry," and take the form of thoroughgoing, serious-minded efforts to learn from our experiences, and the experiences of others, in ways that are critically minded, creative, planned, and intuitive.
- Formal research and everyday inquiry can be enhanced by mindfully and perceptively connecting them with "action."
- "Action research" or "action-and-inquiry" are human activities, and as such, are always affected in ways that can be beneficial, or limiting, by human perception and cognition, by emotions and by one's social, cultural, and historical circumstances.
- Action research and action-and-inquiry can be better practiced, appreciated and understood in the context of human endeavors that are referred to as "science"—and further, these scientific efforts are much more varied and nuanced than the seemingly straightforward procedures taught in most texts on "research methods" and "science."
- Action research and action-and-inquiry can also be better practiced and understood in relation to other intellectual traditions, including human development, social learning, adult education, epistemology, qualitative and naturalistic research methods, and expert knowledge.
- The notion of working toward "transformation" is a more worthwhile, ambitious goal than working for any sort of improvements, insights, or changes. Although resulting "transformations," whether with respect to individual(s), group, organization, community, or the larger society, may be modest and on a small-scale, it is worthwhile to aim for fundamental transformations. That is, transformative action

research or action-and-inquiry has as its intention, to achieve results—insights, questions, actions, and/or changes—which are more than incremental, and more creative than what one would have first expected at the start of one's endeavor.

Transformative action research is not defined by a standardized set of procedures, and yet is not to be done in just "any way," but in ways that embrace some key, critical qualities which are themes throughout the book. These qualities, or fundamental principles, may result in many different, specific types of inquiry. Sometimes an action-inquiry may make a difference only in the life of the person doing the action research, or perhaps only a small change in an organization, school, group, or neighborhood. Other times, it may more deeply and broadly bring about some longer-term change that may affect many people or have a significant impact on a few. An example of fundamental change brought about by WISR students doing action research were to influence a Supreme Court decision, and another was to improve professional practices to prevent child abuse and neglect in an entire state.

End note

1   See also Bilorusky, 2021, chapter 14.

2

PRINCIPLES, THEMES, AND CONCEPTS

As noted in Chapter 1, I initially used the term "action research" in a careless way, as a convenient and simple label, to refer to a rich and many-faceted complex of ideas, methods, and concerns that involve putting inquiry-and-action together. I soon came to realize that I was interested in the role of action research in contributing to personal and/or societal transformation, even if the resulting changes were very modest. I also soon became acutely aware of *how the methods of action-and-inquiry must continually be transformed by our evolving purposes and outcomes.* Consequently, "transformative action research" or transformative action-and-inquiry cannot be conceptualized as a textbook-like definition without becoming a static and non-transformative formula. Despite the emergent and ever-changing nature of action-and-inquiry, there are some key principles and underlying concerns and concepts that provide some degree of form and shape, and that can guide our efforts in transformative action-and-inquiry. This chapter is intended to shed some light on a few themes and key qualities, which will be used in considering issues and methods throughout this book.

All of us can create knowledge

At WISR, we believe that all people are creators of knowledge, and can make valuable contributions. On an everyday basis, many people do "research"—they gather information, evaluate it, form hypotheses or conclusions, ask further questions about their tentative conclusions, experiment by trying out in action what they believe they have learned, then engage in further reflection and re-examination of their beliefs, and collaborate with others to try to make "new" knowledge. Some people do this sort of inquiry and everyday building of knowledge, very well, even if not intentionally and consciously. Also, in some cases we may do this very poorly, for example, by unreflectively acting out ill-considered prejudices and opinions. So, at WISR, one of our especially important purposes has been to learn how we can help ourselves and others—scholars, activists, professionals ,and lay people, alike—to do better research, and to become active participants in the process of doing research to improve our own lives, the conditions and circumstances of others in our communities, and indeed, even ambitiously, sometimes, to work for longer-term and larger-scale social change, aimed at such high ideals as social justice and environmental sustainability.

Some themes throughout the book

Please consider these *recurring themes*, or angles from which to think about the ideas, methods, and issues addressed in this book—*the role of "participatory" in research, the doing of "action research" as an intentionally designed project, and a way of living and learning that is characterized by "transformative action-inquiry."*

Participatory research

Long ago, I came to appreciate that oftentimes the most powerful and successful examples of action research are "participatory action research"—research which engages and involves significant numbers of people in taking leadership roles in the conduct of research that will affect their lives and the lives of others in their communities. I became interested in participatory research, especially because those people who are actively engage in any reality—in any community, endeavor, or circumstances—are well-positioned and informed to study and research that reality, and are also likely to have the commitments and sensitivities best suited to taking transformative action. This is similar to Paulo Freire's perspective on transformative pedagogy for social change (Freire, 1972), and John Dewey's progressive-era philosophy of education for a democratic society (Dewey, 1968; Dewey, 2015). These views point to the value of "participatory action research" and the importance of involving as many interested parties as possible in a collaborative process of action-and-inquiry. Ideally, we should not seek out "research subjects," but rather should enlist active participants in a collaborative process of action-and-inquiry.

Certainly, in many cases, some of the actors in the process will be more heavily and continually engaged, and others perhaps more minimally involved. There is a continuum regarding the extent of participation. At one, ideal end of the continuum, the participants are fully and equally involved in designing and directing the research. At an ethically sound, but less ideal end of the continuum, the researcher designs ethically informed research that protects participants from harm and that obtains informed consent from participants, but where the researcher(s) alone design and direct the actual research activities. In the best case scenario, here, the researchers share their findings with the participants, and try to set in motion constructive follow-up on the research that has the interests and well-being of the participants in mind, and that may later involve the participants. In practice, there are opportunities to do valuable participatory research that is informed by the ideal, even though achievement of the ideal is not approximated. For example, those being researched may still participate in guiding the research and making suggestions about specific methods of data-gathering or questions to pursue, as well as in helping to identify at least some follow-up actions. At the very least, all research should address issues of control, manipulation and abuse by the outside "researchers," as well as take into account the "biases" of those not intimately involved in the social setting which is the object of study.

Doing action research

Doing action research can mean different things to others. It can mean any kind of research that results in action and may simply be acting on a rather perfunctory or superficial gathering of information. Action research may attempt to placate potentially disgruntled employees into feeling that they are being heard by those in authority, or to appease marginalized citizens that their voices are "heard" even if there is no constructive follow-up action. However, these are not the sort of methods or outcomes that are valued by transformative action research. I suggest that with action research we should aim for worthwhile new, even if tentative, insights, especially those that might lead toward improvements in well-being among members of a community, toward greater social justice, reduced inequality, and/or long-term environmental sustainability. Rather obviously, sincere, reasonable people may disagree about the best action and research projects to pursue these values. Still, such values should consciously and intentionally inform any transformative action research endeavor, whether the extent of that effort is small and modest, or enormously ambitious.

Living transformative action-and-inquiry

How can we incorporate this into our everyday lives? Action-and-inquiry can be incorporated into our everyday lives, as we try to be critically minded and creative, and to communicate clearly and authentically, or take other actions, with a sense of purpose. Transformative action-inquiry may impact the qualities in how we live, in:

- how we seek out experiences, and makes observations from our experiences;
- how we go about critically and imaginatively reflecting on those observations and experiences; and
- how we ask questions, make plans, and decide on our next courses of action.

In my efforts to promote transformative learning among people of all ages, and from many, varied backgrounds, I've tried to encourage and enable them to see, and pursue, ways of making action research part of their everyday work and lives. I've seen many instances where people have benefited from learning how research methods could be feasibly adapted to practical, immediate, professional, community, or organizational purposes. Most community groups, educators, and helping professionals can make effective use of research, and frequently that research must be done by action-oriented people, not by professional researchers, if it is to be done at all. In the face of daily job pressures, it is also quite easy to become intellectually isolated, and our imagination and our interest in ideas can easily become stifled by the demands of the immediate tasks before us. Most people committed to community improvement do not have the luxury of stepping entirely outside such demands, as traditional models of research and study tend to require.

Consequently, I have tried to help people learn how to understand some practical uses of research methods during their daily activities. For example, I will suggest ways to increase intellectual stimulation in community-action and work settings, by including regular, scheduled opportunities for stepping back and looking reflectively at the relentless, continuing rush of day-to-day activities. I will discuss ways we can further our continued intellectual development by supporting and collaborating with those around us. In this book, there will be examples of how to make action research methods directly relevant to practical needs of community agencies—such as program evaluations, needs assessments, and long-range planning—reducing, hopefully, our reliance of on outside consultants and "experts."

Instead of focusing exclusively on technical skills and formulas, I suggest that we learn about a broad range of ways in which research can arise out of, and then also affect, our daily lives. Beyond our individual efforts, we can examine ways in which collaboration among individuals and among community groups can help us to arrive at more comprehensive, critically informed viewpoints on the problems that we share. Such cooperative efforts can bring together people from different organizations for mutual benefits, and *develop among us a steadily increasing number of professional and community participants who are knowledgeable about action research, and quite importantly, who can then help to teach others about transformative action-and-inquiry.*

What's involved in trying to be "transformative"

As we pursue our purposes to make a positive impact on the world, in order to be truly transformative, *it is important that we re-evaluate those purposes*, in light of our experiences and latest insights, as well as with regards to our basic values and evolving commitments.

Unfortunately, however, research is often used primarily to justify the status quo, or our own existing goals, or at least to accept, unthinkingly, the assumptions and dynamics underling the status quo. Thus, our action and research may appear to be value neutral and "disinterested" because it embraces values and assumptions that are simply taken for granted. All too often, it is only when our intended outcomes do not fit in with the existing status quo that they appear to be "biased." Many ideas about "science" take the misguided view that scientific research has either has no intended social consequences, or that any consequences will necessarily be "good" ones, so long as scientists engage in a so-called detached pursuit of "pure" knowledge. Fortunately, in the past few decades, many have become aware of how scientific activity is sometimes strongly influenced, for "better" or "worse," depending on one's values, by the purposes and questions (and oftentimes, funding) that guide the research. Research, or "science," is a human activity that is both a product and an important determinant of social-historical forces. *During any transformative inquiry, we must strive to be conscious of the many ethical dilemmas encountered, values and options to be debated, and tough decisions to be made.*

To achieve the sort of "transformative awareness," we must aim to be inclusive, to learn from others and to promote diversity and inclusiveness. This means giving conscious attention to cultural and generational differences, to learn from and address issues of privilege and marginalization, and to recognize and affirm gender diversity. Transformative action-and-inquiry requires that we seek out and learn from those whose experiences and perspectives are different from our own. Then, ideally, with a concern for social justice, our resulting actions and insights may have important value and benefits for those who are more marginalized and less privileged.

By using transformative action research activities as vehicles for continuing, shared communication about what is going on in our professional work, agencies, and our communities, we can often transform and improve our agencies, benefit our communities, and gain new ways of helping one another and each of ourselves, as individuals, to grow and to learn in the process. Potentially, action research methods can be used to explore ways in which we can transform, or circumvent, some of the basic constraints and obstacles, which are faced by most attempts to bring about personal, organizational or community/societal transformation.

In addition, our methods of action-and-inquiry themselves must change, as we further our learning into whatever our inquiry or actions are about. Changing our procedures in the "middle" of an effort does not necessarily increase bias. Transformative action research encourages us to make "quicker" mid-course corrections and revisions in our plans, rather than finishing out the current "study" and having to wait until the "next" study to do it "better." Still, we must let others know how and why we made these changes in our methods in mid-stream so to speak.

Some important qualities of a transformative approach to action-and-inquiry, to be discussed in greater depth in Parts II and III, are that it:

- is exploratory (rather than narrow or habitual);
- is reflective (rather than rote or unthinking);
- promotes engagement (rather than aloofness);
- is inquisitive (rather than disinterested or accepting);
- is collaborative and participatory (rather than disconnected from dialogue and participation with others);
- is emergent (rather than formulaic or mechanistic);
- is concerned with the "bigger picture"—with other theories, readings, larger societal issues and implications (rather than focusing on trees to the exclusion of the forest and the landscape beyond the forest);
- promotes telling and listening to stories and tangible examples (not just abstractions);
- is concerned with human values and social justice (not with so-called value-free research, or with research and efforts which only serve the status quo);

- involves taking one's own experiences and insights seriously, as a basis for thinking, writing, conversations with others, and larger action (rather than relying only on the knowledge from books and the ideas embedded in existing policies and practices within organizations);
- involves looking beyond oneself, as well—as in doing reviews of literature and interviews with others (rather than assuming we can't learn from others, even those whose thinking or purposes we believe to be flawed in important ways);
- involves writing and rewriting in our own voice—to think out loud with oneself, to communicate and share with others, to stimulate collaboration and participation with others, and to refine ideas and strategies (writing is part of an ongoing creative process, rather than an end point or an opportunity to set knowledge "in stone") (Bilorusky et al., 2008, p. 24).

3
BUILDING ON INTELLECTUAL TRADITIONS

The ideas and methods discussed in this book build on several intellectual traditions, and it is important to consider the contributions and relevance of these traditions: the most creative practices of mainstream science, naturalistic and qualitative research in the social sciences, the ideas of the educators John Dewey and Paulo Freire, the guiding metaphor of "script-improvisation," and the Dreyfus Theory of Expert Knowledge. Loevinger's theory of ego development is also quite valuable as is Vygotsky's Zone of Proximal Development.

Thomas Kuhn, the structure of scientific revolutions: "Thinking outside the box"

I have benefited greatly from studying science, initially as an undergraduate physics major. Since then, I have continued to learn from philosophical, sociological, and historical perspectives on science. "Science" is not a fixed, abstraction, but an ever-changing, human, and very social, activity. Science reflects human strengths and limitations, and the methods and findings of science evolve over time. Scientists are affected by:

- the power of intuition and inspiration, and the blinders of poorly managed emotions;
- the biases and the critically minded insights of public dialogue; and
- the discerning qualities, as well as the limiting cognitions, resulting from human reasoning, among others.

One aim of science is to engage people in collaboration that aims to maximize the positive and insight-producing qualities of science, while trying to become aware of, take into account, and minimize the impact of the inevitable challenges and potential limitations that we all face as human beings. So, what is science?

What does it mean in the social sciences? It is important to see "science" as an activity done by groups of people, and by individuals, as a type of human action. Unfortunately, some views misleadingly and intentionally separate "science" from action. In quantum physics, the Heisenberg Uncertainty Principle suggests that we can't separate ourselves from what we are studying. I share the view that we must be conscious and transparent about how our activities of inquiry are connected with the "subject," or realities, of our inquiry. Like many, I, and my colleagues have learned much from the modern-day classic, *Structure of Scientific Revolutions* (Kuhn, 1970).

I first encountered Kuhn's *Structure of Scientific Revolutions* (Kuhn, 1970) as a young graduate student in higher education at UC Berkeley in the late 1960s. At that time, I had come to be very concerned with and even quite critical of the rigidities and perceptual blinders of conventional higher education, and of most all conventional practices in the professions—be they law, architecture, social work, medicine, or physics, the last being my major field of study as an undergraduate. I was extremely interested in learning more about the value of both scholarly and practical endeavors that result from "out of the box" thinking. In reading Kuhn's book, I was struck, as were many others, with how his historical analysis of developments in science, and in scientific and scholarly communities, could also be used to think about developments and challenges in many other professional communities or even among citizens working together for constructive social change. This valuable book is well worth reading, because it can help us in evaluating both the strengths and limitations of ways of inquiring into the matters that concern us.

Usually we learn in school that science is a collection of "facts" or "truths" and that science progresses, somewhat linearly and sequentially as more "facts" and "truths" are added to our body of knowledge. Kuhn's ideas came from his studying, through history, what scientists actually do in fields like chemistry and physics, as individuals and as communities of scholars.

According to Kuhn, science is the history of relatively long periods of time where there are stable plateaus of relatively small changes in thinking. Scientists agree on the dominant theory, or "paradigm," and this agreement enables them to do illuminating "puzzle-solving" which allows them to collaborate easily in using the dominant theory to get "new" information that fills in greater details about "how things work." Quite significantly, however, these periods of stability are punctuated with dramatic periods of crisis and revolution in the scientific community—questions and ground-breaking research are fueled by "anomalies" or data that are "exceptions to the rule" to what would one expect given the dominant theory.

During the long plateaus of what Kuhn calls "normal science," scientists generally agree on the main theory or "paradigm" that they use in identifying what to study and how to interpret what they observe during their studies. Kuhn discusses the value of specific examples which scientists use to illustrate and understand the agreed-on paradigm, and he refers to these instructive examples as "exemplars" of the paradigm. In science classrooms, students are told stories of famous experiments and are given demonstrations so that they may learn the paradigm through an understanding of the exemplars. During the times of stability in the scientific community, the work of scientists pretty much proceeds like clockwork. Scientists may disagree on some details and use these disagreements only to fine-tune the widely accepted paradigm. These small points of disagreement pale in comparison with the strong consensus about the dynamics of the phenomena being studied the scientific community. For example, for hundreds of years, Newtonian physics dominated, and there was widespread agreement, until the revolutions of Quantum Mechanics and of Einstein's General Theory of Relativity. Kuhn studied how these "scientific revolutions" come about, what goes on during them, and how they are resolved.

There are some important lessons for us from Kuhn's historical analysis. First, "normal science" is a valuable, but limited, approach to inquiry, where most scientific activity involves small-scale puzzle-solving. Certain problems are defined as the relevant and interesting ones, and scientists then focus their attention on finding ways of solving these problems—to the exclusion of all other problems. They pay attention to certain kinds of facts, not to others, and make relatively similar interpretations of the phenomena they observe in looking for solutions. As Kuhn observes, during "scientific revolutions" old facts are looked at in new ways. There is a re-study of previously known data, and scientists give attention to data which were previously thought to be irrelevant—either because those data were purposely excluded, or simply not seen as "data" at all.

Some of the processes in the scientific community during the period of "crisis" and "revolution" are:

1. Initially, one or two scientists observe "anomalies" or exceptions to the rule that "don't fit" and aren't explained by the existing dominant paradigm.
2. Sometimes, intuitive insights, such as those made by Einstein, anticipate anomalies that are later observed.
3. As more of these anomalies are identified, a subgroup of the scientific community begins to rebel against the dominant paradigm.
4. As members of a particular scientific community begin to challenge and to ask questions, at first, most others ignore these questions or anomalies, or even strike back against them. Usually, as more anomalies come to awareness, the scientific community is engaged in major debates—the competing sides tend to talk past one another because they cannot even agree on a basis for settling their differences.
5. When the rebellion gets large enough, the scientific discipline goes into "crisis"—this crisis is not just theoretical or epistemological, it is also emotional and political. And,
6. typically, after some fairly protracted period of crisis and conflict, the revolution is successful and most all scientists in the particular field come to agree on a new paradigm or theory, and it is one that combines the insights and scope of phenomena addressed by the previous paradigm, as well as being able to explain and make sense out of the anomalies, in a way that is integrated and coherent.

The new paradigm, or theory, resulting from the "scientific revolution," synthesizes the observations and evidence of concern to each of the warring camps of the two competing paradigms. For example, quantum mechanics has incorporated the insights of Newtonian physics, although physicists are struggling to come up with a "unified theory" that incorporates the general theory of relativity with electromagnetism. This fascinating problem is beyond the scope of this book, but it is an important reminder that even in what many consider to be the "hard" sciences, there are many loose ends and the quest for knowledge is truly unending.

To summarize, the following are especially valuable insights from Kuhn's book that can be applied to developing transformative action research and every day action-and-inquiry:

1. Science is not an abstract thing, but a series of ongoing activities performed by real human beings, with all the strengths and limitations that real human beings bring to their endeavors.
2. Science is a public endeavor, performed by a *community of people in dialogue* with one another—sometimes cooperating, sometimes competing, having agreements and disagreements, sometimes not communicating well with each other, and other times learning a lot from one another.
3. A paradigm is the theoretical perspective that scientists in a particular community use to guide and inform their research and inquiry. The paradigm is useful in facilitating the puzzle-solving of normal science, but it also can limit out of the box thinking, as well.
4. Science itself as an organized pattern of human activities has a sort of structure as well, but the structure, and the process of inquiry, is much messier, more complex, more debatable, less cut-and-dried and not nearly so straightforward and "objective" as what continues to be taught in most science textbooks. Any "science" has periods of unrest, rebellion, and disagreement among the expert scientists in that community.

Why does this matter in the social sciences, and in our endeavors to engage in transformative action-and-inquiry? *Over the years, I have seen how Kuhn's insights can suggest to us some important qualities of good inquiry to which we should aspire.* Specifically, I recommend that we should try to:

1. seek out more productive dialogue with others, rather than less;
2. keep our eyes open for anomalies, or circumstances or examples that are "exceptions to the rule" rather than being blinded by a slavish adherence to one way of thinking.

Much of the value in what Kuhn says can be learned from some questions implied by his book, not just what he states explicitly. What does this suggest to us about the difference between "good" and "not so good" research and inquiry? What do the terms "subjective" and "objective" mean? How can these terms be useful ideas, and how are they oftentimes misleading and based on faulty assumptions about the realities of science performed by real human beings, with all the strengths and limitations that we may bring to our inquiries? The story Kuhn has told us is both good news and bad news for the uses and limitations of theories and paradigms of practice to guide our research and our actions. The good news is that by agreeing on a paradigm or accepted point of view, a community of professionals or scholars have their attention focused on issues, facts, questions, and problems that are often helpful and that they might not otherwise notice. A medical doctor is trained to look for symptoms of certain ailments, for example, and in many ways, this is a good thing. At the same time, the bad news is that the paradigm used by medical doctors may lead to their overlooking certain symptoms, or failing to look for some potentially useful information, not acknowledged by the current professional paradigm of medical practice. Social workers, educators, community activists, policy makers, and people in all fields should be aware of both the "good news" and "bad news" about their use of the prevailing theories, methods of practice, or paradigms.

Kuhn's analysis was based on a study of the most mature and well-established of the scientific fields, such as physics and chemistry. In the last 100 years, and with accelerating speed in the last 50 years, the social sciences have come onto the world's scientific scene. Because of the relative youth of these sciences, researchers in such fields as sociology, psychology, anthropology, political science, and economics, have often assumed a posture of inferiority to the better-established scientific fields. Thus, perhaps, social scientists have often felt compelled to mimic "normal science," which involves seeking the stability and respectability of careful, but not always so imaginative, puzzle-solving and fact-accumulation. In doing so, I believe that they have neglected the more creative side of scientific inquiry, as well as some of the more humane and ethical issues that are involved in any science that takes people and societies as its subject matter.

Consequently, although many texts imply that there is only "one" scientific "tradition," people today, and throughout history have been guided by different ideas about inquiry. In this book, I try to highlight that we always have choices to make about both our overall perspective on inquiry, as well as the specific methods we use. Even the transformative approach to action research may sometimes involve the use of quite conventional techniques of social research, such as, structured questionnaires. Mostly, I will be discussing an overall logic and perspective on inquiry that is quite different from the usual, formulaic approach to research outlined in many textbooks.

Finally, most of the methodological principles emphasized in this book, such as the importance of looking for "exceptions to the rule," are not new, even though they are usually neglected by conventional social research. In many ways, our transformative approach to science has more in common with the working principles of a Darwin or an Einstein than with the popular, commonly stated principles and methods that one might find in most textbooks on social research methods. Most textbook versions of "the scientific method" are much more simplified than the ways in which the most creative and accomplished people have practiced "science."

Qualitative, naturalistic methods and symbolic interactionism

An important tradition in the social sciences is that of qualitative, "naturalistic" approaches to social research, informed by the symbolic interactionist perspective in sociology. George Herbert Mead and Herbert Blumer (Blumer, 1969) were the founders and leaders of this school of thought, and well-known sociologists who have followed in their footsteps include Howard Becker (Becker, 2017) and Arlie Hochschild (Hochschild, 1990; Hochschild, 2012a; Hochschild, 2012b; Hochschild, 2018). These sociologists believe that social *researchers must be actively involved in the social realities, or circumstances, that they are studying*. Participant observation, often accompanied by interviewing, are key methods, where the researcher assumes, in part at least, a role as a participant in the "scene" or circumstances they are studying. Quite commonly, they will interview those people who are the natural, and well-informed participants in group, culture, or situations being studied. Sometimes the interviews may be informal conversations, or at other times, somewhat formal and highly structured. *The researchers are guided by their social values and concerns in deciding what to study, and at the same time, they make a conscious effort to look at things from different points of view*. Oftentimes, they will intentionally seek out participants who may have different roles or different ideas about the social reality being studied, and ideally, they will look for "exceptions to the rule," where people may have different interpretations and things to say about their experiences.

For example, in the 1950s, when studying the culture of medical students engaged in clinical training, Becker (Becker, 1963) formed an initial hypothesis based on his early observations about the motivations of the medical students for pursuing that career. Specifically, he found that most readily stated that they were motivated by the prestige and the earning power of being a medical doctor. So, as a follow-up, to look for exceptions to this theme, he then privately interviewed some students, to see if they would "admit to" any other motivations. He found that many indeed stated to him, something they were reluctant to state in the presence of their peers, that they also had strong altruistic motivations to help people. In the process, Becker painted a more complex, and likely, more accurate, picture of the medical student culture than if he had only gone with his first impressions. Interestingly, in this example, if Becker had done the same study in the 1970s, he might well have first learned of the students' altruistic motivations, and then perhaps later, many students would have also "admitted to" some materialistic motivations as well.

Themes emphasized by the naturalistic approach

The approach and methods of symbolic interactionists in doing such qualitative research emphasize a few, related themes:

- *The researcher becomes heavily involved in their topic/area of study, and becomes very familiar with the lives and experiences of those people who are naturally involved*— whether they are studying marijuana users (Becker, 2018), people who hang out on a street corner in a particular neighborhood (Liebow, 1967), the culture and human relationships in an assisted living facility (Hochschild, 2012a) or people in Louisiana inclined to the politics of the "tea party" and of President Trump (Hochschild, 2018), or even the officers of a major corporation (although it should be noted that powerful people are not so likely to allow others to observe their behavior and circumstances "from the inside"!).

- *The researcher makes a strong effort to understand the perspectives of the people they are studying—how, and why, do they view and experience things the way they do?* Symbolic interactionists take the view that people are influenced by others in deciding what meaning and significance to give to their behavior and the behavior of others, and individuals may also interpret actions idiosyncratically, as well. So, when observing people, we must ask, "what does each aspect of their behavior and actions *mean* to them?" As we develop and articulate our own analysis of what's going on in the situation, we should consciously try to do so in a way that remains consistent with the meanings and experiences of the people involved. Since it is not easy to discern what meanings people give to their actions, we must listen carefully to what people say, and be open to different interpretations of what we hear and observe.
- *Herbert Blumer refers to the process of looking at an idea or insight from many different angles as "inspection."* Blumer likens this process of inspection to holding an object in one's hand and then looking at the object from all sides, and I would add, perhaps feeling how heavy it is, what it smells like, noticing the texture of its surface, and so on. In a similar way, *when doing naturalistic, qualitative research, we try to learn about the "nature" of what we are studying by examining what we are learning from the people involved from many angles and perspectives.*
- *As part of this process, the researcher will quite likely consider alternative interpretations or hypotheses.* To do good research, we must keep in mind that there may be more than one way to interpret what the data are pointing to. We must be prepared to do further research to test out and examine the alternatives, and then, eventually, discuss how and why we believe one alternative is the "best."
- *The researcher will modify, and redirect, their researcher methods as they learn more.* We should aim to use our initial insights to come up with new questions, both questions that we ourselves will be thinking about, as well as questions to ask the people involved in the situations we are studying. We should seek out people to observe and talk with, who are likely to broaden our insights; in this way, we can try to tap into the variety of perspectives and experiences. So, we should actively try to learn about different meanings, different experiences, and perspectives among the group of people we are studying. This is in contrast with those approaches to research that formally define the methods to be used prior to the research, and then stay with those methods, in a misguided approach to not be "biased" by what they study. Naturalistic, qualitative research attempts to allow the nature of what we are studying guide and direct our decisions about the methods we use. Whom should we interview next? Why? What have we overlooked? What questions should we ask, or which people should we talk

with, to not overlook something important? How can we make sense out of information that, at first glance, appears to be contradictory?
- As the researcher comes up with tentative hypotheses or concepts that seem to be useful in making sense out of the varied, and sometimes seemingly contradictory, information and observations, *the researcher will use specific examples and stories to illustrate their concepts.* This approach to illustrate concepts with a variety of relevant examples is what some people call "grounding" the theory. Fifty years ago, Barney Glaser and Anselm Strauss, medical anthropologists, at University of California, San Francisco, wrote the important book, *The Discovery of Grounded Theory* (Glaser & Strauss, 1967). In this book, they suggest that initially one may formulate a theory with only one example or case study, and then proceed to test out and revise that theory as researchers, over time, try to take into account a larger, and more varied range, of examples or cases. *I will later say more about Herbert Blumer's important notion of the "sensitizing concept"—a concept that includes a diverse number of relevant specific illustrations—that evolves and develops as we do further research* and encounter a richer, and more varied range of specific examples.
- *Qualitative researchers, therefore, tend to see all theories as tentative and in need of further development and revision.* A researcher may formulate an imperfect theory, and then, on their own, or with research done by others, attempt to flesh out and test out the theory by becoming immersed in additional situations that are relevant to the theory, and that provided a broader perspective. *Herbert Blumer refers to "exploration" as the process of making conscious efforts to get more varied perspectives and data* (Blumer, 1969).
- *Qualitative researchers often write about their findings by "telling the story" of what they did during the research process, and how they came to their findings. In this way, they try to be transparent about their methods, and potential biases—because in reading the story of their inquiry, we can decide whether, and in what ways, to take our research seriously.* Howard Becker (2017) discusses this methodological approach and suggests that the researcher openly discuss when their insights changed, and what information/data led them to that change. When did they decide to look for further information, and why, and with what further insights, if any? I would add that telling this story is somewhat like what an attorney does in their closing arguments. They tell the jury how and why they have come to their conclusion. How did they weigh the evidence, and what is the conclusion that the evidence points to? Obviously, in a court of law, the attorney is trying to "win" the trial, but the process of communicating publicly, to others, the process of inquiry and how conclusions were then arrived at, is somewhat similar to qualitative research.

Using the above guiding principles, qualitative research aims to look for, and understand the significance and meanings of, the underlying dynamics of whatever social realities or situations are under study. Such research begins by arriving at insights about patterns and themes that illuminate our understanding. Quite importantly, such research then proceeds by paying attention to situational, or specific variations on the themes. For example, as I've learned from WISR alumna, Monika Scott, LMFT, it may be that, generally speaking, when foster youth "age out of the system," they face enormous difficulties, financially and due to a loss of family and interpersonal support. However, there may be variations on this pattern, and if even in some cases, one, two or a few foster youth are able to overcome these difficulties, these variations on the theme, or "exceptions to the rule," may provide us with valuable insights that can be helpful to other foster youth aging out of the system, and to those who wish to provide them with assistance in the face of the support they lose when they become adults. This is the goal of Monika Scott's longitudinal research on what happens to different foster youth, over time, as they move into adulthood. So, the conclusions in her forthcoming dissertation that builds on her Master's thesis will be as much about the details of these "anomalies" as they are about the common themes and outcomes.

So, with qualitative research, one's inquiry identifies themes and variations on themes, leading toward theories. Here, the concepts and the relationships between concepts are not stated merely as abstractions but are also illustrated with a variety of tangible examples that convey the nuances and variety of forms that the concepts and relationships can take. Articulating abstract or generalized concepts and theories in combination with many specific illustrations of the abstractions is what Blumer means by "sensitizing concepts" (Blumer, 1969).

The late Herbert Blumer, Professor of Sociology at UC Berkeley for many years was an important scholar with extremely valuable things to say about the development of theories from observations as the central feature of "better" research in the social sciences. In his article on "What's Wrong with Social Theory?" (Blumer, n.d.; Blumer, 1969), he suggests *a different type of concept—the "sensitizing concept."*

What does a sensitizing concept "look like"?

This kind of concept is contrasted with formal concepts that read much like a 20-word dictionary definition of terms and contrasted with operational concepts which are defined by the quantitative procedure for measuring a concept. For example, psychologists might debate the definition of "intelligence," some saying that it is a single ability to learn and make use of knowledge, and others might say it is a whole variety of different types of abilities or "intelligences." Nevertheless, in using a formal definition, each group, with their paradigm, might try to boil the concept down to a relatively short statement, such as "'intelligence' is really a multi-factor, constellation of different abilities or 'intelligences' that represent the capacity to develop and use different skills and abilities." Such a one or two sentence definition is a "formal concept." An operational concept would define the concept by the way it is measured—so if someone developed intelligence tests in seven different areas, a psychologist who agrees with the "multiple intelligence" paradigm might say that "'intelligence' is not a single entity but rather a combination of seven 'different intelligences' each of which is defined by a particular, seven scale 'intelligence test.'"

By contrast, if psychologists were to take the sensitizing concept approach, they would do extensive observational research in the real world and note a variety of different instances of what seems to be "intelligence." They might use the formal concept as a starting point, but would not stop there, and would try to flesh out in considerable detail what each of seven components (if they continued to have evidence supporting the seven components theory) look like, and how, if at all, those components interact. Although they might make "general statements" and assertions that sound like the formal concepts, they would not stop there. They would look for a *variety* of different illustrations for each concept or generalized statement, and they would continue to look for more and more observations related to the statements, including looking for observations that might not "fit in" with their previous understanding. These unusual observations or exceptions to the rule would be used to revise and fine-tune their concept of "intelligence." In this way, the sensitizing concept is always critiqued and revised by considering new experiences/observations and insights. That is, the sensitizing concept continues to evolve and be refined over time in a continuing dynamic interaction between general "themes" and "examples," between introspection or critical reflection on what we have experienced or seen, on the one hand, and active curiosity and exploration for new experiences and examples, on the other hand.

We might say that *the sensitizing concept embraces a coherent constellation of similar, and yet also quite diverse, array of examples, of situations, organizations, people, and/or stories*. To an extent all concepts, like all words, sensitize or orient us to pay attention to the ideas, experiences, or situations to which they refer. Concepts like "racism," "anxiety," "poverty," "injustice," and thousands more, help us to notice, discuss and inquire into what we "think they are about." The point emphasized here is that by combining the concept with a variety of relevant illustrations of the concept, we may be better sensitized and oriented to what we are trying to learn about, and maybe also, take action about.

There is no one strategy, per se, by which to develop sensitizing concepts, but it does require paying continual attention to data-gathering which involves finding and studying a variety of illustrative examples of the concept, strategy, or theme with which one is concerned. Eliciting stories and looking for a variety of types of evidence as well, are valuable strategies.

Let's consider the concepts of "racial injustice" and "mass incarceration." Here, two concepts may be developed as sensitizing concepts to a significant extent by studying in great detail whether there is a causal relationship between them. And if so what are the *details* of how this relationship plays out? We will better understand the theory if we better understand many, different examples of "racial injustice," and if we know more about the details of what "mass incarceration" looks like. Michelle Alexander, in her book, *The New Jim Crow* (Alexander, 2012), has vividly portrayed not only the concepts of "racial injustice" and "mass incarceration" but also the specific dynamics through which racial injustice has grown and has then led to the growth in numbers of people incarcerated in the U.S. She cites specific studies, statistical trends, *and qualitatively observed and well-documented actions,* that flesh out her theory. The concepts, and relationships among concepts, articulated in her book are good research partly because of the many, and extremely specific, illustrations of how those concepts and relationships operate in our society today. As we learn more about what racial injustice and mass incarceration look like, and as we learn more about how and why they operate the way, they do, we are further developing and improving on the theory put forth by Michelle Alexander. This might include, for example, learning more about the forces that encourage the privatization of prisons, and in turn, how (and whether) prison privatization leads to more African Americans and other marginalized people being imprisoned, and for longer terms. Of course, further research could suggest that Michelle Alexander's theory, like any theory, may be wrong in important ways, or limited in minor ways that still may suggest valuable refinements to the theory.

In the last half of Chapter 11, I suggest beginning directions for developing "trauma" as a sensitizing concept. In particular, I note how the concept of "trauma" has come to be discussed in many different ways, ranging from the results of severe abuse and disasters to the consequences of an accumulation of what has come to be called "micro-aggressions." A briefly worded description of the definition of trauma is insufficient to embrace this complexity, and even valuable indicators like the now, well-known Adverse Early Child Experience Scale, do not by themselves address the complexity and multiple facets of this concept. Developing "trauma" as a sensitizing concept, like the development of most sensitizing concepts, may begin as the efforts of a single person inquiring into a range of instances of that concept. Yet, beyond any initial efforts, it is a continuing process of investigating more deeply and broadly the multiple, and usually varied, specific manifestations of the concept, as well as probing to understand underlying dynamics of cause and effect pertaining to the concept. The reader may wish to skip ahead briefly to read the last half of Chapter 11.

Sometimes a person's "story" further develops a common concept, such as "stigma" into more of a sensitizing concept. This is the case with the recent book, *Another Kind of Madness: A Journey through the Stigma and Hope of Mental Illness* by Stephen Hinshaw (Hinshaw, 2019). In that book, Dr. Hinshaw writes about his childhood experience growing up with a loving father, who for extended periods suddenly "disappeared." He later learned that his father was intermittently hospitalized due to "schizophrenia." He tells this story from both a personal vantage point, as well as from the view of a highly respected and expert academic and professional in the field of psychology and mental illness. In the process, he interweaves specific illustrations of his, his father's, and his whole family's experience with "stigma" and helps to develop stigma as a "sensitizing concept" that is of value to professionals and scholars in the field. This book builds on similar efforts, quite notably Erving Goffman's, *Stigma*, which portrays how the process of being stigmatized has manifested itself with people from many different walks of life (Goffman, 1986). So, ideally, developing a sensitizing concept may begin with one person's efforts in transformative inquiry, but requires the continuing collaboration of many.

In summary, the naturalistic approach to inquiry in the social sciences emphasizes developing research methods adapted to the circumstances and realities being studied. So, rather than having a formal, standardized set of methods and techniques, the researcher must adopt a flexible and improvisational approach. The researcher must still pay careful attention to principles of scientific rigor, including for example, critically evaluating the validity, usefulness, and appropriateness of the data or information that they seek out and pay attention to. Further, they must weigh and critically evaluate what is oftentimes a complex, and even contradictory, array of "facts" and evidence. In doing so, they must disclose to those with whom they are communicating how and why they arrived at their findings and conclusions, and in this way, subject their methods and outcomes of their research to transparency and public scrutiny, which is a key ingredient in any scientific endeavor.

Transformative action-and-inquiry as transformative learning—Freire and Dewey

My ideas about the role of action-inquiry as a transformative force in everyday life, have been greatly influenced by two educators, both of whom were very much concerned with social change—the late Brazilian educator of the last half of the 20th century, Paulo Freire (Freire, 1972), and the well-known United States' early 20th-century progressive-era philosopher and educator John Dewey (Dewey, 2015; Dewey, 1968). Both were strong advocates of learner-centered education and believed that any approach to education must begin by focusing on the experiences of the learner and by seeing learners as active participants. Freire opposed the "banking model" of education that views learners as passive recipients of knowledge from others. Dewey's philosophy of education was that teachers must understand and attend to the experiences of learners. In pursuing transformative action research, it is critical that, like Dewey and Freire, we seek to understand the experiences of others and view each person as an "active agent." Why is this important? First, we must do this to understand them and their social lives well, and second, we must respect others as possible participants in the knowledge-building and change efforts that may grow out of the action-oriented inquiry.

Freire's approach involved him working with groups of people living in marginalized and oppressed communities. He would engage people in dialogue with the purpose of their becoming more consciously aware of their circumstances, and in the process, aim for them to come to see themselves, and others in their community, as having the capacity for addressing and transforming the conditions that were oppressing them. Freire emphasized dialogue and collective action as strategies for action-and-inquiry. He saw his role as an educator to, first, understand the culture and circumstances of the people with whom he would be engaged in dialogue and inquiry. Secondly, he believed that by "posing problems" to others, he could engage them in critical reflection on their oppressive circumstances—that learners would come to realize that there is hope that change can happen, and that they might likely choose to be active participants in the inquiry, and the action, needed to make changes.

In a somewhat less radical way, Dewey saw active learning, and broad-based citizen participation, as essential for creating a functional and democratic society. Dewey was a strong advocate for women's rights to vote, and a humorous story about him was that one day, after teaching his class at Columbia University, he hurried to get to a demonstration in the middle of Manhattan demanding that women get the right to vote. He quickly grabbed a ready-made sign and joined the march, holding high the message, "If men can vote, why can't I?" (from lecture by Professor, James Jarrett, UC Berkeley, 1968).

So, Freire and Dewey promoted approaches to education that were concerned with working toward larger social ideals and values—in Freire's case, the liberation of oppressed people, and for Dewey, the realization of the all too often elusive democratic ideals of the United States.

Dewey believed that educators must challenge and support learners and do so with an understanding of the experiences and viewpoints of the learners themselves. He believed that the aims of education should include helping people to see the world holistically, in terms of interconnections and dynamic possibilities for change. He was against what he saw to be the artificial dichotomies of objective-subjective, end-means, theory-practice, and content-process. I've always especially appreciated his idea that it is important to have a sense of direction rather than a goal. By this, he meant that if one has a goal, one has predetermined exactly where one is headed, but if one has a direction, one begins in that direction, *and* quite importantly, one's direction may change as one learns more, based on one's action-and-inquiry. In this way, action-and-inquiry can be transformative, because we have not prematurely committed to, or fixated on, a specific goal.

Script-improvisation

How did I come to appreciate the metaphor of "script-improvisation" to guide my efforts to engage students in transformative action-and-inquiry? For five years from 1971 to 1975 I was a young faculty member, first at the University of Cincinnati and then at University Without Walls-Berkeley (a small private, nonprofit), and in working with students, I became deeply involved in trying to personalize learning for each student. At the University of Cincinnati, I developed, with another young faculty member there, Dr. Harry Butler, and with two dozen students, an Individualized Learning Program (ILP) in the College of Community Services.

We made a conscious effort to free student learning from the constraints both of pre-packaged curricula with standardized assignments and requirements, and also from contract learning with specific, negotiated learning plans decided upon at the beginning of a student's studies or learning project. The learning accomplishments of students in the ILP were generally 1) meaningful to the interests, purposes and needs of each individual student, 2) outstanding in quality (based on assessment of student papers, community projects, and regular dialogue). *The quality of interaction and collaboration between students and faculty was also greatly enhanced, and the combination* of creativity and collaboration led us to label the ILP's model as one of "an experimenting community" characterized by "script improvisation" (Bilorusky & Butler, 1975).

In analyzing the transformative action-and-inquiry dynamics of learning in the ILP, Harry and I wrote the following:

> ... the nature of the experimenting community is probably best captured by the concept of "script improvisation." The learning process involves a continuing dialectic between script and improvisation. This method avoids learning by exemplar and the rigidities of paradigms. Script-improvisation has direct implications for connecting theory and action, since such distinctions are not inherent in the learning process. The experimenting community differs from mere experience-learning in which individuals, believing they are operating without theory, may impose implicit personal theories or scripts on the world. In fact, this is the pitfall which theories are supposed to overcome. Theories and scripts bring their own pitfalls of reification and overgeneralization. By participating in the dialectic of script-improvisation, individuals learn the process of interaction between theory and action. By continuously examining and constructing scripts and theories in an action context, distortions become apparent. A parallel research methodology may be found in the works of Blumer (1969) and of Glaser & Strauss (1967) (Bilorusky & Butler, 1975, p. 152).

"Script-improvisation" leads to greater effectiveness, creativity, and expertise, as contrasted to on the one hand, not having knowledge or experience with any "script" or theory or strategy at all, or on the other hand, being unable to deviate from and improve on one's scripts. The power of script-improvisation can be observed in many domains of activity—playing chess or basketball, dancing, psychological counseling, teaching, engaging in community activism, or medical practice. Further, script-improvisation can be especially powerful as part of a collaborative activity, as can be seen among a team of people trying to solve an organizational problem, scientific researchers trying to arrive at a new, insightful breakthrough, or a group of jazz musicians having a jam session, among others.

My subsequent experiences as core faculty member and Director of Graduate Studies at University Without Walls-Berkeley further contributed to my understanding of *the value of the "script-improvisation" as a guiding metaphor in open, personalized curricula, aimed to facilitate transformative action-and-inquiry*. In the process, I became aware of the limitations of pre-defined "competencies" as guiding concepts for learning. Although competency-based education, like contract curricula, was designed to free students from the rigidities of conventional, standardized courses, it still imposed subtle, but significant limitations on student learning. Typically, educators defined competencies narrowly, and not as useful guides with considerable heuristic value. So, in practice, competency-based learning was not conductive to transformative action-and-inquiry, because it employed precisely defined criteria to assess student learning, rather than using "competencies" as scripts from which to improvise, and as food for thought (Bilorusky, 1975).

Certainly, the standard "competency-based" approach guides faculty and students in helping learners to achieve some foundational knowledge and skills in their chosen fields, be they engineering, medical practice, or counseling. However, without conscious attention on helping and guiding learners to critique the situational limitations of their foundational understanding, and without developing the skills and motivations to improvise and be creative, learners will not likely progress to higher levels of proficiency and expertise. Creative mastery involves developing expertise that enables one to take a "transformative" approach. That is a central concern of this book, and in the next section, we will see how other intellectual traditions and theories, especially the Dreyfus Theory of Expert Knowledge, provide conceptual frameworks to aid us in promoting transformative learning, and transformative action-inquiry.

Developmental theories for transformative learning—Loevinger, the Dreyfus brothers, and Vygotsky

In trying to facilitate transformative action-and-inquiry among learners, I have become aware of the value of two, developmental theories—*Loevinger's Theory of Ego Development and the Dreyfus Model of Expert Knowledge*. My colleague, Harry Butler, introduced me to Jane Loevinger's Theory (Loevinger, 1976). Then, during the 1980s, I became aware of the stages of expert knowledge and skill development as conceptualized by Hugh and Stuart Dreyfus (Dreyfus & Dreyfus, 1985). Since then, I have become increasingly appreciative of how the Dreyfus Theory can be used in guiding us toward increasingly sophisticated levels of practicing methods of transformative action-and-inquiry that contribute to our greater expertise in our chosen domain(s) of endeavor.

Loevinger's theory of ego development

Harry Butler and I wrote that Loevinger's stage theory uses

> a cognitive-developmental approach to the study of the socialization of [people]. This theoretical perspective suggests the importance of studying interrelations between conceptual arenas which are all too often seen in isolation from each other: curriculum building, human development and learning, social systems and organizations, and visions of [people-and-society]. (Bilorusky & Butler, 1975, p. 146)

Overall, *conventional curricula and many conventional methods of social research* are consistent with Loevinger's *conformist stage*, where people embrace and rely on rules, and wish to find a sense of comfort in very well-defined procedures and standards. At the "next" stage, which allows for a very modest measure of openness and curiosity beyond a strict adherence to rules, there is Loevinger's *self-conscious stage*, which is a transitional stage from conformist to "conscientious." This stage parallels 1) highly structured, but slightly personalized, *closed contract curricula*, and 2) *research methods which are very structured, and pre-defined, but still a bit responsive to the specific circumstances* one is studying and/or in which one aims to take action. From a cognitive and psychological point of view, in terms of Loevinger's stage theory:

> The push for individuality arising from awakening consciousness of inner feelings is appeased by the offering of quasi-individualized education. Meanwhile, the needs for reassurance typical of the earlier stage of conformity are maintained in curricular structuring. (Bilorusky & Butler, 1975, p. 148)

At the next level toward more transformative learning, inquiry, and further ego development, there is the *open contract model* of learning, an approach to inquiry that is consistent with Loevinger's *conscientious stage* of ego development. Action-and-inquiry at this stage evaluates theories and practices to see the situations in which the theories and practices apply as contrasted to those where the theories and practices may not work. In addition, the individual pursuing the action-inquiry becomes emotionally involved, realizing that their actions have consequences that matter to others. As the individual becomes more consciously engaged in evaluating alternative courses of action, they also become more acutely aware of the inevitable uncertainties and complexities involved. Consequently, the individual may sometimes be torn between being assertive and being immobilized by self-doubt.

> The conscientious person is self-critical, strives for goals, is aware of choices, is concerned with improving [themselves], and achievement is important and is measured by one's own inner standards … Conformity at this stage is not to rules or established structures, but to shared or shareable rights and duties. At its best, professionalism typifies this stage. For example, professions strive to achieve sub-cultures which are characterized by reciprocal relationships, shared standards of excellence and ethics, and altruistic responsibilities. (Bilorusky & Butler, 1975, p. 149)

In the discussion of the Dreyfus Model of Expert Knowledge Development (below), we will see how the conformist stage approximates the "novice" stage of expertise, with the self-conscious stage being quite similar to the "advanced beginner" stage, and then the conscientious stage being similar to the stage of "competence" in the Dreyfus model.

Beyond this "conscientious" stage of cognitive ego development, is Loevinger's *"autonomous" stage. In developing the perspective of this stage, individuals begin to embrace script-improvisation* and the value of collaboration and of seeking out others to participate in a sort of *"experimenting community."*

> Loevinger states that this stage is so named partly because one recognizes other people's need for autonomy and partly because individuals are more free of

excessive striving and feelings of responsibility. There is concern with social problems beyond the scope of the person's immediate experience, and there is an attempt to be objective and realistic about self and others ... The autonomous person experiments in [their] continuing search for self-fulfillment, understanding, and justice. Respect for the autonomy of others allows possibilities for collaboration not likely in lower stages, although it is recognized that such interaction can occur in other models ... Rather than separating science and social action, the experimenting community is based on a methodology which integrates thinking and acting (cf. Glaser & Strauss, 1967; Blumer, 1969). Members of experimenting communities are necessarily aware of the unity of the process of learning and that which is being learned. (Bilorusky & Butler, 1975, p. 151)

The thinking and acting characteristic of this stage of ego development, and the related approaches to learning and to action-inquiry, are very transformative and closely parallel the Dreyfus stages of "proficiency" and "expert."

Before discussing the Dreyfus model in detail, some words of caution are in order. Stage models only apply to certain domains of experience and behavior and not to the totality of "who" people "are," so we should not use stage models to "pigeonhole" people. Further, I am only noting some *potentially useful parallels* between three theoretical models—Harry Butler's and my progression of increasingly open curricular models, Loevinger's stage theory of ego development, and the Dreyfus brothers' articulation of a progression of stages toward increasingly expert knowledge and skill development.

In keeping with a transformative approach to action-and-inquiry each of these models, and the parallels that seem to exist among them, are scripts for improvisation. They are not to be seen or used as definitive frameworks to explain neatly and unequivocally human behavior and experience. As this book is aiming to emphasize, all theories should be used as "scripts for improvisation," as potential starting points for further inquiry-and-action. Furthermore, any one of us is likely to be operating at "more than one" stage at any given time. So, in some ways, I may take a rather conformist approach in some aspects of my life, conscientious in other ways, and once in a while experience and behave in some of the ways characterized as "autonomous" by Loevinger. Using the Dreyfus model, I may be "novice" in some area of knowledge or skill (for example, in my case, in drawing or painting with watercolor), "advanced beginner" in other areas (e.g., use of the Google Education Suite), "competent" (in driving an automobile), "proficient" (as a ballroom jazz dancer), and perhaps getting close to "expert" (in using action research).

With these exceedingly important qualifications in mind, before discussing the Dreyfus model further, consider Table 3.1 (below) of very approximate parallels.

Dreyfus brothers' Theory of Expert Knowledge and Skill Development

The advantage of any theory in emphasizing certain patterns or key themes is also its Achilles' heel, in that, if we are not careful in using the theory, we may lose

TABLE 3.1 Parallels between Dreyfus Theory of Stages of Expert Knowledge, Loevinger's Stages of Ego Development and Four Curricular Models

Stages	1st	2nd	3rd	4th
Dreyfus/expertise	Novice	Advanced beginner	Competent	Proficient and expert
Loevinger/ego development	Conformist	Self-conscious	Conscientious	Autonomous
Butler/Bilorusky—curricular models	Conventional/Pre-packaged	Closed contract	Open contract	Experimenting community and script-improvisation

sight of other complexities and nuances that are deserve our attention. Indeed, I value the Dreyfus model partly because it points out that, *at higher levels of skill and knowledge, beginning at their proficient level of skill and knowledge, one must perceive, act, and think in ways that cannot be boiled down to any neat, definitively articulated theory or paradigm*. This is very much in line with Polanyi's view (Polanyi, 1966) that *we can know much, much more than we can put into words and make easily accessible to others. Therefore, our personal knowledge is much more extensive than the "public knowledge" that we can easily share with others*. Certainly, public knowledge is also very important, and as noted earlier, Kuhn has learned through his scholarship, that science is based on the public knowledge of an articulated paradigm, that is agreed upon by scientific experts in a particular field.

Somewhat paradoxically, the Dreyfus model is an effort to put forth as public knowledge how people progress to greater levels of expertise, even when that expertise cannot be neatly shared as public knowledge. Furthermore, my affinity for the Dreyfus model is not simply because it is consistent with what I like to say to others about action-inquiry, but more because it resonates with what I have experienced, and have come to appreciate and sense quite deeply based on my many years' of experience with dozens and dozens of colleagues and others from many walks of life, and with different interests and passions. The Dreyfus model is an exceptionally good "public knowledge" articulation that approximates some important features of my personal knowledge.

According to the Dreyfus Theory of Expert Knowledge and Skill Development (Dreyfus & Dreyfus, 1985; Dreyfus & Wrathall, 2016), someone operating at the novice level relies on specific rules, just to begin to function in that domain. This may be called a "cookbook approach" where one must follow precise directions, out of a lack of experience and understanding. At the "advanced beginner" stage, specific, *approximate* indicators can be seen in how the learner approaches action-and-inquiry in that domain of growing expertise. For example, the person will:

- demonstrate an understanding of more than one's perspectives and/or strategic approach within that domain of knowledge or skill development;

- demonstrate that that they can apply and adapt ideas and/or principles of practice, situationally;
- show that they can look beneath the surface of the way things might appear at first glance, and by identifying circumstantial exceptions to the rule;
- be motivated to seek out further ideas, practices, and deeper insights; and
- actively reflect on what C. Wright Mills referred to as the "Sociological Imagination"—looking for the connections between the specific experiences of individuals and bigger picture societal dynamics (Mills, 1961).

At the "competent" stage, specific, *approximate* indicators in the person's approach to action-inquiry are that they will:

- demonstrate knowledge of at least several theories and principles of practice within that domain of knowledge or skill development;
- be able to critically examine theories and principles of practice, to identify the circumstances in which each is most likely to be useful and valuable, given the strengths and limitations of those theories and strategies of practice;
- be able to engage in conscious and deliberate planning and make critical comparisons of alternative courses of action, and will identify and explain the relevance of their recommended plan of action;
- show an awareness of the inherent uncertainty, complexity, and subtlety in using such theories and principle; and:
  a. identify uncertainties and dilemmas faced by competent professionals in the field;
  b. identify possible practices and directions for inquiry that take into account those uncertainties and complexities.

At the "proficient" stage, specific, *approximate* indicators of the approach to action-and-inquiry are that one will:

- identify strengths, weaknesses, and uses of several theories and practical approaches within their area(s) of expertise and demonstrate that they can use more than one perspective;
- be engaged in inquiring into, and then formulating, ways in which some of these theories and practices can be improved through the use of informed experience and critical reflection, and by a more holistic appreciation of a multiplicity of varying circumstances, contexts, and impacting variables, that is, the individual will be able generate ideas and/or proposed practices that demonstrate a holistic perspective involving a variety of situational considerations and variables;
- show that they can gather data that they then use in analyzing the variable impact of situational factors;
- as part of this holistic appreciation of a multiplicity of varying circumstances, contexts, and impacting variables, demonstrate that they have learned not just to rely on general principles, but also can articulate, test, and revise concepts

and proposed strategies and practices through stories and case studies, accompanied by reflective analyses; more specifically:

a. be able to identify concepts and insights gained from their research, not in abstract terms, but also coupled with a rich variety of examples that they use to understand and to illustrate the complexity, situational variability and nuances of the concept;
b. demonstrate that they know how to use a "discovery of grounded theory" approach to develop possible theories and/or practice approaches, drawing on data from specific cases, stories, and/or practical experiences.

One moves beyond the level of "proficient" to "expert" through a long, and continued, process of gaining more and more experience, and does so, with a transformative approach to action-and-inquiry. Over time, the expert can take action, and inquire further, guided by their "intuition." This includes understanding theories and paradigms of practice, in ways that are increasingly nuanced. The experience of the expert in their domain of expertise is that most of the time they are actively engaged in further script-improvisation. Each improvisation leads to a more "expert script" which may or may not be conscious. The expert's sense of what they know is deep and strongly discerned, and it is usually much more than what can easily be put into words or reduced into a theory. However, the expert may provide valuable guidance to others by trying to put what they know into words, and formulate as a theory, or set of concepts and principles. Still, without some specific illustrations or stories about their principles, it is difficult for others even to begin to appreciate nuances in the concepts.

Vygotsky's Zone of Proximal Development (ZPD)

In *Mind in Society: The Development of Higher Psychological Processes* (Vygotsky, 1978), Vygotsky defined the ZPD as "the distance between the actual development level as determined by independent problem solving and the level of potential development as determined through problem solving under adult guidance or in collaboration with more capable peer" (Shabani, 2010, p. 86).

Vygotsky's concept of the ZPD (Zone of Proximal Development) is a valuable way to think of how to challenge, and collaborate, with others so they (and in many cases, "we") can be assisted in learning what they (or "we") are ready to learn, but can't quite yet learn without assistance. That is, we can aim to help others, and ourselves, to build on what they/we already know, and engage them/ourselves in the next domain of challenges on their/our path toward greater expert knowledge and practice. This is one of the ways in which collaboration is of critical importance as a key ingredient in transformative action-and-inquiry.

Vygotsky's theory of development and his concept of "Zone of Proximal Development" (ZPD) are very valuable in understanding how and why "readiness" to develop further should be combined with intentional guidance and support.

ZPD refers here to areas, or ways, in which a learner is not yet capable of acting capably or learning on their own. They may be "close" to having a certain capability or competence. However, without guiding help from someone more capable, and/or without the opportunity to learn in an "optimal" situation—one that is challenging, but not too challenging, and also supportive—the learner may have difficulty in progressing or developing their capability to the "next level."

Consider the example of a learner who is an expert professional, and who may design, with guidance from a mentor, an action research project, related to a learner's area of strength (e.g., further developing expertise and knowledge as a somatic therapist) while also addressing a limitation (e.g., gaining insights and experience as an educator of practicing therapists). So, the learner's area of greater strength and expertise becomes a sort of supportive bridge for them to develop in an area where they have less expertise. Further, the learner's mentor or colleague has the role of providing "challenge" and "support" that are "just right." In addition, or alternatively, the learner's mentor may help them to find, or design, a set of circumstances that will help the learner to use their knowledge (in this case as a somatic therapist), to practice, experiment with, and evaluate strategies for educating other therapists about what they know.

As much as the expert therapist may know as a therapist, they do not yet necessarily know all they need to know to help others to learn what they know. But they might be "close" to being able to do this, if the faculty mentor can guide them, can help them to learn from and use what they already know, and/or if they become engaged in transformative action-and-inquiry in conducive circumstances that help them to extend themselves and be engaged in trying out and learning about how to use their knowledge, now, in the role of "educator of other therapists." In this regards, the competent or even expert therapist, who is perhaps only an "advanced beginner" at educating other therapists, is pursuing a learning project within what Vygotsky would refer to as their "Zone of Proximal Development" with regards to learning how to educate other therapists. They are benefiting from the "social learning" from and with their mentor, and/or from and with the situation in which they are trying out their hand at educating other therapists. Methods of transformative action-and-inquiry can aid them in consciously extending their expertise as educators, in this example.

Furthermore, someone who understands many of the principles and methods of transformative action-and-inquiry can be "their own mentor," or at least have a sense of what to do, in order to seek out or create the circumstances in which they can learn within their ZPD. Continuing with the same example, the qualities that the learner who is a proficient therapist brings to their learning task, that is the challenge of educating other therapists, can provide a facilitating "bridge" for them to develop from an advanced beginner in educating other therapists and then become a competent, or even perhaps eventually, proficient or expert educator of other therapists.

Indeed, anyone who understands, or better yet is accomplished, in transformative action-and-inquiry, will have a sense of what to do to become more competent in their "less advanced" area of knowledge. Knowing about transformative action-inquiry, they may well seek out collaboration with others who are more expert in their "less advanced" knowledge domain, and/or they may very well design an action research project where they can gain practice and learn more in this area, and do so with a consciously designed evaluation of their efforts, to learn about what works and what doesn't work. In the above example, they may perhaps learn that they need to reformulate their initial learning outcomes planned for those therapists whom they are trying to educate further about somatic therapy.

Potentially, in their expert role "as a therapist," and with the benefit of an understanding of transformative action-inquiry, this person has served as a guiding colleague for themselves "as educator of other therapists." Their greater expertise and knowledge as a therapist provide a Zone of Proximal Development for the less expert educator, and their learning in this Zone of Proximal Development might be further enhanced by support and guidance given by a mentor or colleague. *As a general strategy, we may often apply this particular transformative approach of social learning in our lives, by seeking out collaboration with others who will help us to build on our strengths while also engaging ourselves (and/or others) in the next domain of challenges on the path toward greater expert knowledge and practice.*

The Dreyfus model, as well as Loevinger's theory, may also suggest ways in which we can collaborate with others in addressing the challenges we encounter on the way toward "greater expertise." For example, to make the transition from "advanced beginner" to "competent," the learner may benefit from guidance and support in finding meaningful ways to become emotionally invested in the outcome of their efforts, whether in an internship, or as another strategy, through intensive study of various scenarios in which they can envision themselves to be committed. This might also include simulated role-playing with fellow students. Such experiences enable the learner to become engaged in conscious, deliberate planning of their strategies and practices, and to develop know-how in long-term planning. "Competent" learners will have opportunities to become "proficient" if they are challenged by colleagues and mentors, or through experience, with concrete instances in their domain of study which counter the normal pattern or accepted theories. To become more expert in this way, a learner should be guided to consider an array of various circumstances and theoretical perspectives, in order to develop a holistic perspective that engages the learner in actively searching for nuances and complexities, and then wrestling with how to make sense out of it all.

In summary, my understanding of, and appreciation for, uses of action research methods, and engagement in transformative action-and-inquiry, has been informed by several intellectual traditions:

- Kuhn's insights about the structure of scientific revolutions;
- the qualitative research methods promoted by symbolic interactionists and those who have articulated the value of "grounded theory";
- the socially progressive and learner-centered, transformative educational views and methods of Paulo Freire and John Dewey;

- the developmental perspectives of Jane Loevinger (on ego development) and the Dreyfus brothers (on developing greater expertise); and finally,
- Vygotsky's insights about the value of social learning, of collaboration, mentoring, and optimal challenge in powering transformative learning.

Emotions matter in research

In the next chapter, we will examine the interconnections between research and society. First, it is quite relevant to consider the interplay of emotions and research. This interplay is more inevitable and complicated than the usual exhortations that we should "keep our emotions out of research."

Our emotions may aid inquiry and they may impede inquiry. Enthusiasm and curiosity tend to aid inquiry, as does a mental attitude of being able to "tolerate ambiguity." Deep, persistent, continuing, and transformative inquiry tends to be messy. The observations and data that we encounter may be contradictory and inconclusive. Emotionally, it is much better to learn to live with such messiness than to err in the direction of trying to arrive prematurely at a neat or definitive conclusion. When Loevinger discusses the mental orientation of those whom she would describe in terms of "conformity," she points out how their preference for feeling "comfortable" fits in quite well with simply following rules and generally accepted norms. People whom she would characterize as "self-conscious" have become comfortable with the idea that there is a multiplicity of possible views on most any matter, and this enables them to "progress."

With any progress, however, there are new challenges, and those of us for whom self-conscious is an apt approximate characterization may become so emotionally fascinated with the myriad of possibilities that we are not so motivated to make choices and commitments among the options. In many ways, each succeeding developmental stage brings new emotional strengths and new challenges. Those of us who are often "conscientious" in Loevinger's scheme are very much aware of our responsibilities and the importance of making the "right" decision. So, although we are now motivated to make choices, our awareness of many options may at times may be immobilizing, because we are so afraid of making the "wrong" choice. The Dreyfus brothers discuss this in talking about the stage of "competent," and Benner's research (Benner, 2001) on students in the nursing profession supports this analysis.

As we move beyond the conscientious stage, we oftentimes become more at peace with our decisions, but this does not necessarily remove us from any emotional conflicts, doubt, and stress. As we become more attuned to larger issues of "justice," as well as our deeply felt emotional connections, including love and commitments with the especially significant people in our lives, we still have strong feelings, uncertainties, and doubts. We can learn to live with these feelings, but this does not necessarily make our lives easy. In these many ways, and more, our emotions are very much part of any transformative action research effort, just as they are of course very much part of our lives as human beings.

Emotions are also key if we are to be able to collaborate with others, to learn from and with others. Collaboration is something that we should aim to do whenever possible, partly because as the saying goes, "two heads are better than one." Also, collaboration is valuable, because action research, or indeed any sort of effort to improve our lives, the lives of some others, or of the larger world must ultimately involve others. Collaboration will be most fruitful, if we can nurture within ourselves, and with others, a sense of respect for one another. Further, transformative inquiry is facilitated if we can develop and embrace a sense of humility, along with a certain amount of self-confidence, as well. We are more able to do worthwhile action research by cultivating our emotions and being mindful of the strengths and challenges found in our emotions. *As you read through the various chapters in this book, try to keep in mind the question of "how do emotions come into play, for 'better' and for 'worse' when doing this type of action research?"*

Kuhn's stories of the drama, and what some scientists may even experience as the melodrama, of scientific endeavor underscores how science is a social and very human process. Others such as Hazen have graphically demonstrated how *science is made up of emotional and political conflicts among scientists, as well as intuition, engaged curiosity, and many other human dynamics that are quite varied and full of the complexities and uncertainties of life* (Hazen, 2005). This reality is contrasted with the seemingly mechanistic, precise, dispassionate, and emotionally detached methods of observation that are presented as essential and unbreakable rules and qualities of scientific inquiry to novices reading books on research methods in the social sciences. What we get in most texts on research methods is the "cookbook" approach to doing research that may be a good first step for novices. However, this is a but clumsy first step for those who would aspire to become expert researchers, either in the natural or social sciences. To progress beyond the novice level, we need a lot of experience trying to do research, as well as critical reflection on what did and didn't work. Further, we can benefit greatly from the sort of deeper insights provided by scholars discussed in this chapter who have delved into complexities and subtleties in the domains of research methods, science, and expert knowledge.

Certainly, there are important reasons that novice learners best begin by being taught simple rules. Further, the development of new knowledge and improved practices are not aided by people's ill-considered biases and emotional reactions. All of us have some emotional reactions and button issues, whether they are recent and situational, or left over from many years of living life. Still, *the commonly stated rules of "dispassionate" inquiry have unfortunately grown to mythological proportions in our society.*

It is valuable that the deep, and careful analyses and observations by scholars such as Kuhn, Blumer and the Dreyfus brothers can help us see and understand how and why systematic inquiry and the development of expert knowledge is not such a simple, dispassionate, linear process. As I noted when considering the insights of the Dreyfus brothers, even though we can sometimes be impeded by our emotions, this is no reason for us to aim to rid ourselves of our emotions. First, it is impossible to do, and otherwise we would be kidding ourselves. Second, *sometimes emotions, as well as our idiosyncratic experiences, may actually aid the development of knowledge and expertise and be invaluable qualities of inquiry, as is especially the case when we progress to the Dreyfus stage of competent and beyond* (Benner, 2001).

Just as emotions are fundamental to all human endeavor, including science and research, so are society, and the culture, groups, and institutions of our society. This will be the focus of the next chapter.

The value and limitations of intellectual foundations—culture, gender, generation, and privilege in transformative action-and-inquiry

As I will discuss in the next chapter, inquiry and research are always informed, for better and for worse, by the values and perspectives of the society in which we live. I believe that more than is the case with many intellectual traditions, the ones discussed above, do "transcend," *to some extent*, the biases and limitations of any society. On the one hand, Kuhn's history of science is a history of Western science, and at the same time, his perspective reveals how "science" in this Western tradition has always been practiced in ways that sometimes reinforce the biases of the scientific community, and at other times, critique and even transform the assumptions of the scientific community, which then results in "advances" or transformations. Kuhn provides us with a perspective to keep in mind in critiquing the limitations of any paradigm or theoretical orientation.

Blumer, and other symbolic interactionists, guide us to seek out actively and consider new experiences and perspectives beyond our own, which is important if we are to work toward transformative inquiry-and-action. In this way, we can try to go beyond the limitations of our own generation, culture, gender, and circumstances of privilege and/or marginalization. Still, these things do matter. It matters who we are; our life experiences and identities very much shape how we pursue inquiry-and-action. Yet, we can aim to go beyond our limited experiences and personal views—by seeking the wisdom, insights and perspectives of others who are different from ourselves, and even ideally, by collaborating with others who are quite different, in some ways at least, from us.

If I had been born 50 years later, I might have benefited from different intellectual traditions—quite possibly some of those discussed above, and also, however, from some others that are based on the perspectives of people representing more marginalized groups, because of their culture or gender identity, for example. As a young adult, I did learn to keep in mind, and look for how systemic and "bigger picture" dynamics impact us immediately as well as over the long-term. I gained insights from Marcuse and Fanon, for example (Fanon, 1967; Wolff, Moore, & Marcuse, 1969). Furthermore, I would have benefited from having sooner been introduced to the ideas of bell hooks, critical race theory, and Audre Lorde, among others (hooks, 1994; hooks, 2003; Lorde, 2017).

Still, the intellectual foundations I have used to inform my approach to action research have helped me to broaden my perspective. In particular, they have informed me of the benefits of collaborating with, learning from and reading about the perspectives of those who are younger than myself (and years ago, with those older than myself), who have very different cultural experiences, who have different gender identities including sometimes a more fluid and non-conforming sense of "gender," and who are less privileged and more marginalized in ways that I can only partly comprehend and appreciate. I am very aware that the authors of the books and articulated intellectual perspectives who first shaped my ideas were men, and mostly not at all marginalized men and raised in European or European American cultures. Important exceptions to this were Paulo Freire, Frantz Fanon, and Jane Loevinger, who was one of the first American psychologists to realize the importance of studying and learning from the experiences of women and girls. I have tried to keep in mind that any intellectual foundation must be used as a *starting point*, and not as a "container," for my inquiry-and-action.

When I was "coming of age," my peers and I would note how "our generation" was different from the older generations. Still, I knew I could learn much from those older than myself, and at the same time, I benefited from the new insights, or at least the more emphatically articulated and practiced commitments, of "my generation." Today, there is much that I can learn from the millennial generation, and I am consciously aware of this, if for no other reason than I take seriously learning from my 22-year-old twins, each of a different gender. Unlike my generation, millennials are painfully all too aware of the climate emergency; and in the U.S., even "middle-class" millennials no longer take for granted that a career will be a secure basis for employment. As a young adult of my generation, I soon came to the realization that a career, in the traditional sense, might not be so meaningful, so I carved out my own path. However, despite being raised by a single mother under very modest economic circumstances in the 1950s, I never was worried that I might be underemployed, much less unemployed, unlike so many young adults today. In my 20s, many of us in "our generation" (which was actually the title of a periodical from the 1960s) were very aware of U.S. imperialism and the oppression of third world people in the U.S. and around the world.

Still, with each passing decade, the depth and extent of the marginalization of people throughout the U.S. and the world has become more and more apparent, and arguably, more and more severe and pronounced. Such awareness has not always resulted in transformative change, but it is probably at least a pre-condition for major transformations. Further, I have seen how, over time, there has been an increased awareness of the many forms of "able-ism"—of how people are marginalized based on different physical abilities or their particular neuropsychological abilities and styles. A member of my family, and quite possibly the most intellectually gifted one, has had to endure, and then overcome, the stigma of a learning disability—having been seen by many teachers and others as "less than" until finally after years of persistence and resilience, as well as some good fortune, having "shown them" that they were wrong. Perhaps, not surprisingly, she has become engaged in inquiry on the complexities of the plight of youngsters, facing special challenges, including those characterized as having "early onset conduct disorders" (Bilorusky, N, 2020). Also, my wife works with the developmentally disabled, and fortunately, laws and practices are gradually, even if still quite inadequately, addressing injustices pertaining to able-ism—and this sort of consciousness needs to inform transformative action-and-inquiry.

Having the good fortune to have been involved with the very diverse group of faculty and students at WISR since 1975, I have learned much from and with people from many walks of life and from many cultural backgrounds, facing different challenges, including sometimes severe circumstances of oppression and marginalization. I have seen how they have adapted and used action research to further deepen their own perspectives, and to pursue their interests and passions. Although transformative action research by itself does not guarantee a multicultural, inclusive perspective, it often can support and aid broader and deeper understandings.

I cannot easily put into words the enormous value and impact of my good fortune to collaborate with so many different people, and for so many years. In the process, I've learned much from others, trying to identify as best as I can with their circumstances and challenges, as well as learning from their insights and talents. When collaborating with someone, I try to listen carefully and attentively to what they are aiming to accomplish and learn about the problems they face. Only after trying, at least, to somewhat put myself in their role and circumstances, can I then modestly raise some questions and make some tentative suggestions about how we might together proceed. And of course, since I may have my own agendas and purposes, I try to share them openly to see if my colleague feels ok about joining with me in pursuing those.

In other words, functioning at WISR and trying to practice transformative action-and-inquiry, has provided an approach and well-functioning context for mutually respectful and transformative collaboration. In the next chapter, I will discuss more explicitly how our perspectives, derived significantly from our societal circumstances, shape, in ways that can be sometimes helpful and other times limiting, how we approach action-and-inquiry.

4

RESEARCH AND SOCIETY ARE INTERCONNECTED

In this chapter, I turn our attention to thinking about some of the ways in which research—the questions, methods, and findings of research projects—is strongly influenced by the larger society. How are research, the goals, and methods, impacted by the prevailing values in the society, by the interests of various groups who have the power to influence what is studied? Similarly, the larger society is oftentimes influenced by research. For example, many years ago, attitudes, and even advertising laws, were dramatically influenced by research which demonstrated a strong connection between cigarette smoking and cancer. Before that, such restrictions were staved off by research supported by the tobacco industry that "somehow" found no cause for concern. Indeed, every day, there are studies which are used to argue for one cause or policy position.

One recent study funded by the Koch brothers, who are strongly opposed to "Medicare for All," found that over 10 years the cost of "Medicare for All" would be 32.6 trillion dollars! On closer examination, other economists noted that buried deep in that same study was a finding that Medicare for All would likely save $2 trillion dollars or more, over that same period (Nichols, 2018). Such research is far from dispassionate, with advocates of various positions sponsoring or citing different "findings"—with some research funded by groups like the Koch brothers who advocate for free market capitalism and insurance company profits, and others doing research to advocate for health care as a right and for elimination of insurance company profits as a way to lower health care costs. Those with special interests can frame their research methods to influence the findings.

Consequently, it is critical that, in evaluating any research findings, we examine the methods used, the assumptions made, and the interests, and values of the people who conducted the research. As noted above, critically minded and careful attention to details finally raised serious questions about the Koch brothers-sponsored research. Most recently, a few months later, research reported in the peer-reviewed medical journal *Lancet* indicated that "Medicare for All" would provide health care for *all* Americans and do so at a savings of $450 billion per year (Galvani et al. 2020).

My discussion of these competing research findings regarding the cost of "Medicare for All" is *not* to suggest that all research is equally biased or flawed, but rather that we must be aware of possible, hidden agendas behind research studies. Furthermore, even with well-intended research, there may be unexamined assumptions and flaws, some of which may be influenced by larger societal forces that shape our questions, purposes, and views about what constitutes meaningful, relevant, and accurate data.

The purpose of this chapter is to deepen our awareness of the place of research as a social institution in today's U.S. society, and the ways that this increasingly powerful institution affects us in community research, leadership, and service endeavors. None of this is to discount the possibility of trying to do solid, fair-minded, and painstakingly careful research, and action research. Instead, we must think about how research is an important and potentially politically and socially powerful endeavor.

Research as a social process

(Revised and updated from an earlier paper with Dr. Terry Lunsford.)

Research is often talked about as if it were an activity aside from society, looking at the world instead of in it, "observation" as distinguished from "participation" in social processes. It is not. This discussion is designed to raise for our consideration some of the ways in which research itself is very much a social process, and to consider some of the consequences of these facts.

Researchers as participants, research as participation

Whatever our place and work in society, we all participate in it—by our occupations, our community work (or lack of it), the attitudes we hold and uphold to others, the ways we spend our time and money, the net results of our work. Research is an important part of such participation, especially so today.

Producing new knowledge is a major industry, today, with its large corporations, its own economics, its professionals and managers, its public relations, its marketing strategies. It commands large government contracts, foundation grants, and fees from business corporations and labor unions. Verified, "scientific knowledge" and its applications are major commodities—patented, bought, sold, publicized, admired, feared, possessed as instruments of power. Whole bodies of knowledge, from spacecraft engineering to new medical technologies to studies of economic trends to human behavioral science and engineering, and artificial intelligence, have their specialized experts, their political constituents, their training programs, their secure places in large, complex organizations. Distinguished scientists, such as Nobel Prize winners, or the "discoverers" of new drugs and artificial organs, are accorded a kind of personal authority and deference once reserved for priests of religious orders, thought to have privileged access to supernatural revelations.

Humans, it is often said, are coming into more control of their world and of human life, and so are approaching (dangerously?) closer to the status of gods. The major instrument of that approach, whatever we may think of it, is science—research, the deliberate and systematic pursuit of knowledge according to the so-called "empirical method." Thus science, and research more broadly, are of immense consequence in society, affect it powerfully every day of our lives, and involve their practitioners in a kind of social participation that is too often overlooked.

As researchers, ourselves, we may not ever come close to the Nobel Prize, to a major breakthrough in medicine or physics, even to uncovering a significant new "truth" about human actions in our communities. Still, we are participating in society, nevertheless, when we do research. The processes I am calling inquiry, or action research, involve to some degree deliberately new and special kinds of actions on our parts, and we ask others to act differently, if only to cooperate with us in letting us formulate research problems, gather data, interview them and evoke new ideas from them, organize these facts and present them to others, and call for new decisions based on new knowledge.

Simply by calling our activity "research," we evoke from others and ourselves a special imagery about what we are doing and not doing. To many, research implicitly raises expectations of numbers in tables, of computers and statistical tests, of turgidly written reports and reasoning that is difficult to follow. To others, it implicitly means impersonal intrusion into the lives of others, useless conclusions understood only to the researchers, and an outsider's lack of understanding about the daily lives of those they are researching. None of these are necessary characteristics of research, or of science, but they fit many examples of research as it is practiced in our universities and our communities today.

Besides being a part of broader social processes—such as the ongoing politics of everyday life in a community—research is itself a social process. Researchers are people, who eat, love, sleep, have needs and motives, combine in social groups, help each other, fight, get jealous, change, become inspired by ideals, feel work-pressures, and do most of the other things that all of us do. The scientific norm of so-called "disinterested" inquiry, which strives to get rid of "bias" in reaching conclusions, has had as one of its unfortunate side-effects to obscure these everyday facts about scientists as people. Scientists try to avoid bias, but they don't succeed, ever … completely; and most of the time, it's a matter of degree. It depends on the viewpoint from which we look at the bias; and it also depends on the purposes to which we put our conclusions. That doesn't mean there is no point to it. The scientific process, and inquiry searching for generalizable truths, have long ago proved their importance and power in our lives. But the image of passionless and value-free and pristine-pure detachment of the laboratory scientist has been misused and misunderstood to obscure the homely realities in an extremely simplistic way, which we should aim to go beyond.

One little-understood part of the scientific process is that science is not the actions of individual, "great men" (all too seldom envisioned as "great women" or "great people") who invent from their genius minds great new ideas and then embody them in magic inventions which they patent and sell to General Electric. Science is in good part a cultural process, meaning that all new "discoveries" rest in part on the general level of knowledge shared in the culture in which the scientist lives, and thus, these breakthroughs rest on the common, shared understandings of many alert, knowledgeable people in that society. Individual scientists do seem to have special abilities, and/or motivations, as well as special access to the knowledge-stores of their society, and these advantages probably do help them to be the ones who come up with discoveries and breakthroughs. Furthermore, societies seem to differ in the degree to which they support scientific institutions, such as colleges and universities, and research labs and discussion groups, among people wrestling with scientific problems. But that shouldn't allow us to overlook that all knowledge, including that kind we call "science," rests on the common knowledge base of the society in general. All scientists "stand on the shoulders" of the rest of us.

Science, and all research, is also social in the sense that it is historical. It involves a lot of people over time, criticizing each other's research, disagreeing with one another, challenging other people's evidence and conclusions, attacking assumptions, arguing for entirely different statements of the problem, trying to see the thing more clearly, trying to get closer to "the truth"—sometimes over years, decades, even centuries. That is why the image of the lone inventor, or great scientist, who arrives at some new conclusion, is somewhat misleading. Very few, if any, conclusions are ever proven by a single study or scientist, or even by a whole scientific career. Bodies of knowledge, which become accepted and useful in a society, are the products of very complicated, social-historical arguments in which many people engage. And, as we know from Thomas Kuhn's work on scientific revolutions, these arguments change radically over time, as old paradigms (theoretical models) lose their usefulness, and new ones emerge which appear to be more valid and productive at the time.

Consider this example. For centuries, Newton mechanics worked very well; it helped people to build all sorts of machinery during the Industrial Revolution for example. However, the more we developed the ability to look far into the night sky, and the more we moved toward serious examination of the interactions of particles within atoms, and not just the atoms themselves, the more scientists began to wonder about some possible limitations of Newton's theories. Einstein formulated ideas about theory of relativity, including the interconnections of space and time, and the "curved" rather than straight line nature of these interconnections. His theoretically developed ideas were later confirmed by observations. At about the same time, in the decades immediately following some of Einstein's initial insights, a different critique, noting the limitations of Newton's theory, led to quantum theory, and in particular, the notion of the "uncertainty principle." That principle, somewhat overly simplified, states that at the subatomic level, especially, we cannot precisely specify the behavior, or even the fundamental nature, of these subatomic waves/particles. These two new insights, which over time were increasingly supported by observational data, did not completely invalidate Newton's theory. Rather, they articulated more pointedly the limitations of Newton's theory. That theory can still be used quite well for building bridges and machines, and for playing pool on pool tables. However, it cannot be used so well if we are studying the expansion of the universe or the path of light over millions of light years, nor be used to study the goings-on at the subatomic level.

Social positions and perspectives of researchers and others

Some social scientists like to emphasize that each of us has a position, or really a number of specific positions in society, and that these affect the ways we see the world in very basic ways. A parent, for example, has a definite place in their family, which is different from the place of her children, no matter what their ages and learning. They treat others in certain ways, which go with that position—wipes their noses, urges food on them, gives unsolicited advice, supplies them with money, hugs them, cries, or fusses over them. They don't do the same things to the parent, at least, not in the same ways and to the same degrees. In this sense, a family is a "social structure," with its parts and their interconnections, and parents are in one part, children in another. These realities shape each person's actions, and also the ways they see the world. The parent tends to worry about things the kids don't; for example, whether they are wearing enough clothes to keep warm. They, on the other hand, think of things the parent doesn't, such as the utter worthlessness of life if they can't have the approval of their current group of friends. In the same ways, researchers and other people who are involved in research have their own, differing social positions and their attitudes are to some degree shaped by those positions.

If you work in a big university department, for example, you may have the position in society called "professor," or the one called "research assistant," the one called "clerk," the one called "graduate student," or any of several others. You will feel pressures to act certain ways, depending on which of those positions you hold. You may not like, or give in to, those pressures, but you will usually be aware those pressures exist, to act in purposive, deliberate ways, at least most of the time. You will be expected to talk in a fairly precise way, using at least some of the special terms of the department's academic discipline; to speak with respect of people who are considered the expert practitioners of that discipline; and to avoid belittling certain kinds of research methods used in the discipline, for example. These are ways of acting—and, implicitly, of thinking and feeling—that your social position in that department, and the contacts that you have with other people there, pressure you to adopt. If you do, it will feel easier to you than if you don't; and if you don't, you will very likely seek out other people with whom you can compare notes, and talk about how stupid it is that people in that department act that way. In other words, you will find another social group, in which you can hold other social "positions," and cooperatively build an alternative social version of the right ways to act, think, and talk.

If you work in a commercial research lab, other pressures will be felt in your daily work—to honor the profit motive, for example, or to sneer at "ivory-tower academics" and to admire practical, down-to-earth, applied research that has an immediate, visible effect on the world, and quite likely that can result in a substantial profit. The pressures will be there, wherever you lodge your research efforts. If you work in a community organization, it is most likely that you will find some people around you who have spent some time in a university setting, and who have some of the attitudes mentioned above that they have brought from that academic setting. But you may also have some friends and co-workers who think that "ivory tower" research is all pretty useless, and who admire applied work, as many do in commercial laboratories. And, you may have co-workers who don't think much of research of any kind, whether their personal experience has led them to suspect and fear research as a weapon used by people essentially hostile to down-to-earth, community purposes, or just because they don't know much about it, and don't see that it has much usefulness in doing the jobs that they think are important, and that need doing right now.

If you wish to use the kinds of action research methods that I am advocating for in this book, it can be vital to your doing good research in your school or community organization that you learn how to get the good will and support of your co-workers and constituents for doing action research. To do this, you are advised to learn something about their attitudes and feelings toward research, and how their experiences have led them to see research in the ways that they do. How much do they really know about it? You will need to help them to understand that there may be valuable, alternative versions of research that are distinguished from outsider-run, un-involved, studies that they may have previously experienced. It's also a good idea to think, to yourself, about your own ideas and feelings about research, how your social experiences, including formal schooling, have led you to think as you do, and how some of the versions of action research discussed in this book can fit in, or not, with your work in your organization, profession, or community. You might consider giving some thought to these matters, and then discuss them with others with whom you could collaborate on an action research effort.

Researchers and research organizations as different

One of the most important parts of the social process of research is its organization. Mostly, in this country, we tend to think of individual people, of "persons," as the entities that are really real in human life, and often see social things, groups and institutions, as "merely in our minds." After all, we can change laws, or rules, or even abolish whole governments or corporations or research groups—at least, in theory we can. In practice, however, these social entities have stubborn persistence, whether specific groups tend to like them or not, and "social change," even the reform of important parts of organizations, is much harder than we sometimes wish it were. The reasons for this are complex, but the point is that these social entities—organizations, for example—are very real. They are there; most of them do not change very rapidly, and their existence has very clear consequences. That is, a group of people gathered on a football field without a leader or without long-term relations among them may be called a crowd, or even a mob, or a group. But if those people are divided into leaders and followers, those with more and less authority in the group, into people with different jobs, if they say they are united by common purposes over a period of time—these and other things we can think of are some of the signs of what we call a "team" or "organization." They are mostly interconnections between people, rather than only characteristics of individuals, themselves. These interconnections are very real, in the sense that they are consequential, and have effects that matter.

Besides the broader pressures mentioned above, working in a big organization, for example, involves getting support—like a salary, and research funds for paper and computer equipment, or advice from colleagues or instructions from bosses. You will receive support, and demands, depending on how you experience it, for what you can study, what methods you must use, and what tools are available to you. You will likely find yourself meeting and talking with some people, and not with others. In a research organization, you will probably talk with those in your specialized research group, who share a common task, not talk with just anyone in the whole organization, at random. Your social life and your work will follow patterns, and those patterns may be shaped in good part by the organizational structure and processes of the place in which you work.

Most organizations with which we are all familiar tend to be organized very hierarchically, meaning that there is a vertical relationship among the people working together, so that some people give orders to others, to those "lower" down, and don't get given orders by them. It doesn't have to be that way, but it is one way of keeping things orderly, and many people seem to resist operating any other way. So, hierarchies keep being re-created, all the time, in organizations that try to operate in other ways. This kind of order, obviously, makes a lot of difference, because it gives some people, usually a few, a lot more power than others. It also directs people's research efforts to some specific purposes, and not to others. It has been said of Ernest O. Lawrence, the famous UC Berkeley chemist, that his most important contribution to science was not the discovery of plutonium, but his creation of the first organized research group on a major university campus. Whatever you think of that, it makes the point that organized research, especially in physics, chemistry, biology, and technology, have helped to revolutionize the way science is done in this society, and have made science a much more powerful tool for those who have access to directing it, and to setting its purposes, and shaping the content and access to the training that scientists receive.

Organized research groups today usually involve some combination of hierarchy (bureaucratic bosses and giving of orders to subordinates, within written rules) and what is called "collegiality" among professionals. Collegiality generally means more equal relations among people, who respect each other as competent, thinking persons, with certain areas where each knows more than the others, and who need to discuss things with each other periodically, in order to pursue the solutions to their problems.

This chapter, and the entire book, is not aimed only at helping people who consider themselves professional researchers, although such people could well benefit from learning about these methods. Here, the focus is on helping a variety of people to learn about methods of action-and-inquiry that may be used to bring about valuable societal and organizational changes, while also promoting their own growth and learning.

This book is especially valuable for people who see themselves as professional or community leaders, or activists, or who plan to be, people who aim to try to change their organizations or communities for the better. Indeed, people from all walks of life might join together to form action research teams and cooperate with each other actively, and get the benefit of the insights that are so often monopolized, today, by the big research institutions and their specialized experts.

The kinds of action research discussed in this book are designed to be done by non-professional researchers, who are engaged in doing rather than only studying, and who want to use their research for transformative improvements, large or small. Working in a community group or school faces you with many different tasks and imperatives not encountered when working in a research lab, and properly so. The question is how to organize your research in your community agency, school, or professional or community group, so that you can define its purposes and methods as collectively as possible and can involve people in cooperative ways. This means helping everyone to think about, how can those affected understand what is being done with them and to them, and how can they share their biases, and their results, openly among the people whose lives they may affect?

In this book, you are invited to think about broader issues that might come up, in pursuing action-and-inquiry that matters to you, when you think of research explicitly as a social process, and how it is very much affected by the way it is organized. For example, what difference do you think it usually makes if research is done by the people who will be using the results, instead of having it done by outside experts, who come in for a short time and then go away? How will it affect the research questions asked if the people who formulate them know the agency or the community from the inside? If they are not specialists in research or social science? What kinds of cooperation between specialists and non-specialists, between insiders and outsiders, between decision-makers and information gatherers, do *you* want to set up in action research that *your* group does? There are many such questions that are worth thinking about.

Research that serves specific social interests and values

Just as research has its places in society, is socially organized, and affects other social processes, it also serves specific interests and values. Depending on the kind of research—the content of the questions being asked, the kinds of answers and data that are sought out and accepted, the ways the conclusions are drawn and the results interpreted—it may help some groups much more than others. It may help to keep presently powerful people in power, or it may help to change power relationships. It may raise questions that give new groups a chance to be heard, or it may tend to keep the voices of those groups muted and muffled by current orthodoxies. In other words, information and the resulting interpretations aren't nice, neutral things, always beneficial in the short and long run, equally available to all groups in society and equally useable by all. They can be shaped to serve to some degree the purposes that we aim for them to serve.

Saying that doesn't mean that research is just a tool of power, that research is just special-pleading and advocacy, in the senses that those terms are often used—as if to distinguish research from the pure search for an unbiased truth. Inquiry as a process—if we do try to find out honest facts about the settings we are examining, and if we do try to build an attitude of finding and using truths among people in a community group—can help to move that group or community away from factionalized, purely contentious, narrowly selfish ways of dealing with problems. Action research can help to build much more mutually respectful kinds of discussions of shared problems. Many of the methods and qualities discussed in this book can provide ground rules, and attitudes toward discovering facts, that guide and shape our approaches to the work we do, and the ways we formulate, critically evaluate and transform the purposes we want to pursue together. Those possibilities are inherent in an transformative approach to action-and-inquiry, which respects the world the way it is, even as we don't fully understand it, and then aims to help us build common understandings on which we can act together.

However, this doesn't mean that all groups have the same goals, or, in the short run, that we can sit down and work out shared goals and methods for working together. It's hard enough, just doing it in a neighborhood or a community organization that already has a lot of common experience with which to work. So, you shouldn't be unaware, or ashamed, if you intentionally aim for your action research project to serve some specific social change purposes that your group defines as important. Further, you should be ready to go through some hard, though probably very stimulating, discussions with each other to think through how to pursue those purposes with your inquiry.

"Science" often is used, today, as a vague label that gives prestige to a narrow agenda that someone is pushing, perhaps in influencing people to comply with that agenda. People may use the term "science" partly perhaps because of its long-time opposition to "magic" and "superstition," and to mysterious processes often misused to fool and exploit people. Nevertheless, "science" as a label can itself also be misused and misunderstood. One example is when one assumes that any so-called scientific advance is in a good direction. Even if some good possibilities do come from a new scientific discovery, such as a new drug, the side-effects may take a longer time to show themselves, and most discoveries will have such side-effects.

So, we need not reject or accept any result as good or bad merely because it is called "scientific." Instead, it is important for us to see what the many effects are going to be, and then evaluate the accomplishment on its own merits. As probably is obvious by now, we think this involves a good bit of understanding of what "science," properly understood, is all about. The transformative approach to action

58 The foundations

research is one way of practicing "science" that tries to make it more understandable, and more available, to all of us who are trying to bring about social change in the direction of improving lives in our communities.

Consequently, I am suggesting that we be reluctant to equate "science" with simple formulas and techniques. "Evaluation," for example, has long been a popular buzzword in community work. It has its real uses. A lot of us know generally what it means, and it may involve our raising questions about what we are doing, and to compare our actions with standards or other practices, or to criticize what we are doing and talk about it to others. However, there are many superficial and simplified approaches to evaluation that have been much misused by professionals who sell it to community groups, by bureaucratic agencies and for funding sources who want a "scientific," or externally defined, basis for their funding/defunding decisions. Many people are under pressure to justify their agency's legitimacy or funding by demonstrating that they can meet "objective" standards of performance. Chapter 2 of the companion book, *Cases and Stories of Transformative Action Research* (Bilorusky, 2021), will include a more detailed discussion of "evaluation." How can we take a transformative approach to program evaluation? How can evaluation impact various groups, for better and for worse? How can those most affected by evaluation play key roles in designing and conducting evaluations?

In conclusion, just because so much of what is called by the name of "science" may seem foreign and technical, and may all too often misused against us, we should not reject it and give up "science" to the "scientists." *Science as we (and many others) understand it is a special version of abilities and understandings that we all have, as human beings. It is a precious possession of all humans who want to participate in it. It can be reclaimed, at least in part, from the big research labs and academic departments that now dominate it. Seeing it as a social process, and as an important part of society, can be a step in that direction. Collaborating with each other in reclaiming science—that is, acting together socially—is very much worth our efforts.*

Historical developments in social research and its underpinnings

(Revised and updated from an earlier paper with Dr. Terry Lunsford.)

A conventional discussion of the Western history of research or inquiry might begin with a study of Greek philosophers, with a study of Socrates, Plato, and Aristotle. This Western history of research might proceed through the Middle Ages, and consider Copernicus' observations of the motions of the sun, the earth, the planets and the stars, and his resulting theory that the earth is not the center of the universe. This history might comment on the conflict between this view of the universe and the prevailing belief, based on religious dogma, that the earth is the center of the universe.

The historical developments most influential on science in the United States in the 1700s were those of the enlightenment-era philosophers of the 18th century and their social impact, including the use of their ideas by leaders of the American and French Revolutions, such as Thomas Jefferson. This philosophical school of thought emphasized the importance of the "scientific method" and the use of human reason in achieving what people then thought of as human progress and social justice. Our standard historical analysis might go on to consider the rise of the German university in the 1800s, for the German university was in many ways the model for the contemporary graduate school and research institute in the U.S. The German university emphasized the importance of specialization in particular fields of study, as contrasted to the interdisciplinary and broad-reaching study of many previous Western scholars, and indeed, the German university initiated the idea of dividing an institution of higher learning into various different academic departments to aid specialized research.

Then, in the 1860s, the Land-Grant Act in the U.S. provided for the establishment of state universities and colleges, including many of today's state universities and the old A&M colleges, as a way of aiding the development and westward expansion and colonization of the U.S. These colleges were created to provide pragmatic, technical assistance in such areas as agriculture and mining, and other fields of economic importance. The contemporary U.S. university is, in many ways, a synthesis of this pragmatic approach to research and learning, with the interdisciplinary liberal arts college, the religious college, and the ivory tower ideal represented by the German university (Veysey, 1992).

The above paragraphs sketchily outline the beginnings of what would be a rather standard, Western history of research. But the standard histories overlook or de-emphasize many other important considerations. In my view of research, research is a basic activity, which is as old as humankind. Research is sometimes aided by written analysis and communication of ideas from one person to another, and from one generation to another. But research does not require writing—people can engage in research by trying to make sense out of their everyday experiences, by sharing their experiences and thoughts with each other, and by passing down oral histories of wisdom on the significance of these thoughts and experiences.

Little, if anything, has been written about the research methods of so-called "primitive" people—i.e., people who did not have written histories, or who lived in hunting and gathering societies. Yet, there is undoubtedly much we could learn from the research methods of our distant ancestors. Such an endeavor would be challenging and difficult, but very illuminating if we could find out something about the everyday research methods of peoples from other times and cultures. Related to these long overdue critiques of IQ tests as a way to define the concept of intelligence, we might have asked much sooner, "has 'intelligence' been an idea embraced by all cultures?" Perhaps other peoples have managed to make sense out of their experiences without having to use this concept at all. If so, it would be important to understand more about the social circumstances and methods of daily action-and-inquiry which led them to give greater importance to other ideas, and less importance, or no consideration whatsoever, to concepts we may take for granted.

Our ignorance of the methods of inquiry used by our distant ancestors is paralleled by the consistent exclusion of histories of non-European cultures in those books claiming to be a "history of ideas" or a "history of science." This narrowness in commonly distributed history books contributes to our ignorance and to racism and other forms of social injustice. For example, how much is commonly known about the Mayans' development of the concept of zero, and of the inquiry and social/cultural circumstances surrounding their development and use of the concept? For those who wish to learn more about some of the many scientific breakthroughs and advances made in Africa, Asia, and Latin America, you may wish to begin by going to the following website: https://hssonline.org/resources/teaching/teaching_nonwestern/

It is important to consider such historical issues not as a matter of academic or esoteric interest, but because a historical perspective can enrich and deepen our understanding of our contemporary circumstances. Research, and indeed all forms of human inquiry, may often influence the course and direction of a society, and conversely, social/cultural conditions shape and influence human inquiry—for example, the ideas considered, the way experiences are interpreted, and the uses of these interpretations.

In significant ways, many new insights are the results of social/historical forces, that is, the results of our social circumstances, and the experiences, values, and perspectives our social circumstances encourage. Even if we oppose the values of the dominant society, the very act of critiquing and opposing dominant social forces points out that society has played a role in producing ideas and research, for our historical conditions have provided the problems and issues that we have chosen to confront.

For instance, in the book *Social Amnesia* (Jacoby, 1985), Russell Jacoby points out how "social amnesia" is a prevalent problem, for not only is there planned obsolescence of material products but also of ideas. Commonly, we believe that "new" ideas must be better, so we are all too prone to be uncritical in grabbing hold of any new fad. In the process, we may lose much of what was insightful and valuable in "older" ideas. Jacoby's book illustrates this trend through a consideration of socially uncritically thinking which characterizes some trends in the field of psychology in the latter portion of the 20th century.

Consequently, those of us involved in any particular sort of community effort—whether working on affordable housing, trying to improve the education of our youth, or working to address the climate emergency—might benefit from a consideration of the historical circumstances, which have led to changes and emerging practices (or lack thereof) in our area of concern. What are the social and historical origins of the kinds of community efforts in which we are involved? To what extent were local efforts shaped by larger societal forces? Were local efforts a reaction against some injustice or social problem which was part of larger historical trend? Are we repeating some of the errors that others made many years before? What can we learn by studying other societies, the nature of their social injustices and problems, and the strengths and weaknesses of their efforts to address those issues?

In her book, *The Shock Doctrine*, Naomi Klein (Klein, 2014) provides many examples of how, during times of crisis and in the aftermath of these crises, powerful segments of the society, those with interests primarily in expanding their profits and control, will use these opportunities to extend their power. One such example is the privatization of schools, and the resulting loss of some public accountability, in New Orleans, in the aftermath of Hurricane Katrina. Supposedly this privatization was going to address the inequities and ineffectiveness of public-school education. Instead, it has made things worse, as Klein documents in her book. So, today, during the coronavirus pandemic, we might learn from some of the history lessons provided by Klein.

The pandemic is bringing into the open, much more vividly, the inequalities in pay and working conditions in this society, the health disparities that weigh especially heavily on African Americans and other marginalized groups, the absence of a well-prepared, well-funded public health system, and the need for universal, publicly controlled health care. Yet, as Klein has recently pointed out, powerful business interests in the tech sector of the society are using this crisis to push for our turning over control to them, rather than just trying to make better use of technology. To be sure, we need technology more than ever during these times when it is well-advised that many of us should try to live in near-quarantine situations (Klein, 2020). Nevertheless, an important unasked question should be, how do we make more extensive and improved use of technology while still providing for public control and decision-making about all this? And, if we are to make such decisions, what can we learn from history to guide and caution our efforts? Do we run the risk of focusing on the "obvious"—the need for better and wider spread use of technology—without asking harder questions about what do we really want for ourselves and one another to improve our lives and the society? As Klein implies in that recent article (Klein, 2020), do we just want to have more widespread use of technology for teaching children, or do we want smaller classrooms and better staffed schools with nurses and art teachers added? Do we perhaps want better use of technology, and especially better use of technology that is guided by the experiences of parents and teachers, and not directed so much by those who make and distribute technology for a profit? Critical thinking and historical and contemporary analyses are of the utmost importance, here.

Further, we may critically examine the uses of research in recent history. How have various research methods contributed to community problems and social injustices? Have certain methods given misleading information or undue emphasis to certain social issues with the detrimental effect that other information, ideas, and problems have been ignored? Can we identify some instances in which research efforts seem to have had a constructive impact, either on a local level or on a larger, societal level? Consider, for example:

- research on the concentration of wealth in this country;
- research on the relationship between cigarette smoking and lung cancer;
- massive testing of students and use of achievement tests for college admissions; and,
- research on the causes of the climate emergency.

To promote discussion and transformative action-inquiry, we might well ask ourselves the following questions about various contemporary research efforts:

1. What are the social/historical forces which motivated and/or shaped these research efforts?
2. How did these research efforts affect people in the society, and help to create certain changes in the society as a whole and maybe even in the direction of history?
3. Did these research efforts mobilize any activities or further research in opposition to them?

Concluding remarks

In so many ways, our society and our culture, *and especially those groups and people with the greatest power, influence and privilege,* may significantly influence, and distort, our inquiry in ways that we may not always readily appreciate. Action research cannot realize its transformative potential without a consistent and continual awareness of the challenges involved in addressing these biases. These biases are not merely "academic" matters that influence our "research conclusions," for they impact our lives and our society, and especially the lives of those who continue to be most marginalized and least privileged people in the society.

PART II

Methods of action research—steps in the process

This part of the book describes and discusses specific methods of action research, organized primarily by the four "steps" in the process, from what typically happens at the beginning of a project, asking questions and defining the problem to be studied to what is often seen as the end of the project, communicating with others what has been learned, and "then" taking action. However, it is important to add that, with the transformative approach discussed in this book, the following steps in the process of research need not always follow the usual conventional sequence, but may continue to interact and interweave with one another throughout the process of action-and-inquiry:

> **BOX 1 STEPS IN THE PROCESS OF ACTION RESEARCH**
>
> 1. asking questions (Chapter 5),
> 2. sampling (where to seek data and information) and the actual data-gathering (Chapter 6),
> 3. analyzing data (Chapter 7), and
> 4. communicating what has been learned during the research and collaborating throughout the process (Chapter 8),
>
> as well as, of course, with action research, the important, additional step of taking action!

Action may happen before, during and/or after the research, and ideally, we should remain conscious of all three options. The actions, before we intentionally begin, still contribute to that research effort. During the research project, our actions are likely to lead to further insights and inquiry. Finally, we will use what we have learned to take action, and even to do more research.

Chapter 6 is largely about what some people call "data collection methods," but it is more than that, because the transformative approach to action-inquiry reminds us that this approach is not only about action research "projects" but also more broadly and deeply, about how this can become part of our everyday lives. And, in our life, we continually have experiences that are very much like "data collection" and "sampling" to select sources for our data. Therefore, I also call our attention to becoming more conscious about where our ideas and "facts" come from, and the value of "broadening our experiences."

Chapter 7 may seem like it is supposed to be about "analyzing the data" to get our "findings" in a research project. And again, it is about much more, how do we make sense out of our experiences, how to we weigh and judge evidence? These are processes which are important in research in particular, and more generally, in our lives as a whole, as well.

Chapter 8, which includes extensive discussion of the strategies and importance of collaboration, is one of the most important chapters of the book. Good collaboration greatly strengthens any action research project, improves and deepens what we can learn throughout our lives, and is critical for mainstream scientists doing cutting-edge research.

There is a fifth chapter in Part II, Chapter 9, that is devoted to quantitative research methods. Included is a brief, general overview, and discussions of the strengths and limitations of quantitative methods. Further, that chapter provides some, specific instruction to help the reader gain at least a "qualitative" understanding of quantitative methods of graphing and computations. Finally, we consider the uses and misuses of statistics and how to use quantitative information with qualitative data.

5
ASKING QUESTIONS

The importance of asking questions

(Revised and updated from an earlier paper that was initially written with collaborative assistance from WISR faculty member, Vera Labat, MPH.)

Asking questions is an essential feature of any formal research project, action-oriented or otherwise. Most research begins with questions, and, despite the popular notion that research ends with conclusions and findings, it is perhaps more significant when research projects "end" with the formulation of even "better," more interesting questions for future research, thought, and action.

Generally, the first step in designing an action research project is to decide on the main questions, goals, and/or problems that will serve as the initial guide(s) for your project. I say "initial" guide, because a transformative approach to inquiry and action research acknowledges that as we learn more through action-and-inquiry, we may well revise our questions or goals, or redefine the problem we are trying to solve.

A number of years ago, WISR received a contract from a Community Redevelopment Agency to conduct a major study of the needs of low-income elders living in downtown area of a major U.S. city, and to assess the adequacy of the whole gamut of services that were available (or not so accessible) to meet the elders' needs. When the representatives of the Redevelopment Agency first met with us, they emphasized that they wanted us to look at the entire range of services—food, transportation, safety, recreation, and much more; however, since millions of dollars had been recently spent on building low-income housing, we needn't bother to do research on housing needs. When we embarked on our research, as we recommend to anyone doing research, we still asked not only some specific questions, but also many very broad, and open-ended questions—to the elders and many services providers and advocates with whom we met. Interestingly, they frequently volunteered the view that the single, biggest unmet need for many low-income elders living downtown was for better, safer, and affordable housing! So, despite the Redevelopment Agency's initial definition of the problems to be addressed, we changed course and decided to do a lot of further, very targeted, investigation into the lack of access to housing. The details that we learned are interesting and beyond the scope of this book. However, let's just say that we learned many important things about why and how a great need for low-income housing remained, contrary to the assumptions and directives of Redevelopment Agency staff. This important lesson illustrates the critical value of being open to changing the problem statement and questions that direct one's action research effort, as more information emerges.

In addition, when students at the Western Institute for Social Research (WISR) are about to embark on a thesis or dissertation, those of us on the faculty usually start by suggesting that they think about what few questions are important to them that they would like to "learn more about" in the course of their thesis or dissertation research. We say, "learn more about," rather than "answer," because very often if we come up with questions that we consider possible to answer we will be less imaginative and ambitious than if we come up with the questions we deeply care about that we know, consciously or unconsciously, that we may not be able to "answer" so easily. In other words, it can be quite important to just pursue questions, even if we don't conclude or answer any of them in a clear-cut fashion. This is contrary to the conventional notion that a good research project formulates a thesis statement, or hypothesis, to be proven or disproven.

Certainly, building evidence in strong support or refutation of a thesis statement can be an important part of the ongoing process of inquiry. For many purposes, "proving" or "disproving" a hypothesis can be of critical importance. For example, one could hypothesize that a new drug is effective in combating an illness and can do so without side-effects. This is a legitimate, and potentially valuable, way to formulate one's research, even though the "answer" is still seldom a definitive "yes" or "no," but rather a qualified statement such as "yes," in 95% of the cases it is effective, and the negative side-effects are not so serious and are relatively rare. Still, many conclusions based on the traditional hypothesis-testing model are even more qualified than this.

In many cases, and for many purposes, coming up with conclusions or evidence which build a "conclusive" or "strong" case may be less important than formulating provocative, meaningful, engaging questions which push us to probe beneath the surface of what we know, and to learn things which may ultimately be genuine surprises and breakthroughs, for ourselves and for others. Oftentimes, meaningful questions can be raised to follow up on the uncertainties resulting from the hypothesis-driven research. For example, if a drug is not effective in 5% of the cases, medical researchers might well make progress by asking, "why not?" and then do research on this 5% to learn more. Or, they might well try to learn more about the incidence of negative side-effects, and the underlying dynamics of these side-effects, in order to produce a drug without such side-effects. Whether one is doing "new" research on a topic or following up on a large body of existing research, asking questions that are critically minded and imaginative is extremely important.

Asking questions

As discussed in Part I, T.S. Kuhn (Kuhn, 1970) points out that "normal science" is like puzzle-solving with an emphasis on answering questions that are taken for granted. In contrast, scientific revolutions involve coming up with fundamentally new ways of looking at things and are usually promoted by asking completely different questions than have been asked before.

Beyond the important role that asking questions plays in formal research projects and scientific endeavors, whether in the natural sciences or social sciences, asking questions are important to life. Indeed, the transformative approach to action research blurs somewhat the distinctions between inquiry in everyday life and inquiry in formal research projects. It is important to ask questions all the time, and also, sometimes we may intentionally formulate a "project" to be "extra-systematic" in framing questions, gathering evidence and/or reflecting on experience and action, and generally using our questions to guide our efforts to learn more through action-and-inquiry.

Let's consider some important questions about asking questions:

- Where do questions come from? From a sense of discomfort? curiosity? Or?
- Why ask questions? That is, why is it important to ask questions?
- What kinds of things can be accomplished by asking questions? For example, perhaps we can get clarification about what we already think? Do they help us to listen to others and learn from them? Maybe they can help us to enlarge or enhance our own creativity? Illuminate our thought process? Enable us to be playful in inquiring about things we care deeply about, because we don't have to keep, or go along with, anything that we come up with, if we later decide it doesn't make sense or doesn't seem to be of value?

We can learn a lot by sharing with one another some of the memorable questions that have come up for us in our day-to-day lives. We might well find out from others about questions that they are asking in conjunction with their community or professional projects, or on which they are about to embark.

To aid your investigation of "asking questions," here are several "thought exercises" that you might consider doing:

- Can you think of a question a child has asked recently?
- What do you notice about the question-asking that children engage in, as compared with the question-asking of adults?
- Can you think of a question somebody recently asked that you have no idea "where it came from"?
- You might intentionally notice questions others ask, and ones that pop into your head, and then reflect on what this might tell you about "question-asking"?
- After reading a good book, or thinking about a stimulating TV show or movie, you might reflect on the question-asking that is explicit and the question-asking that is implicit in that work. Then, ask yourself, "what are the ingredients of the question-asking?"

We can do these thought exercises of question-asking on our own, and we can oftentimes get even more out of it, by later going through this process with others, by sharing our thoughts about question-asking with one another. We could discuss what each of us see to be some of the qualities of "good" vs. "not-so-good" questions.

Thinking about question-asking is important, because very often we get bogged down in the essential routines of work, family life, survival, and our own habits that have evolved over time. Such routines are not all bad, and indeed, they may be essential in important ways. However, they may sometimes detract from asking "good" questions. Perhaps children learn rapidly because so many things seem new and not so routine. In graduate school many years ago, I was very struck by an article by the ego psychologist Robert White (White, 1959), who observed that children demonstrate quite strongly what he termed a "competence motivation." That is, young children are not generally satisfied to have everything orderly and neatly worked out. They seem to have a rather unrelenting motivation to create challenges and to "make problems," and I would add, "raise questions," for themselves. This seems to help them to develop a whole host of competencies and in relatively short periods of time.

Asking questions about your community organization

(Revised and updated from an earlier paper with Dr. Terry Lunsford.)

As we work in community groups and other organizations, day in and day out, many things about them became all too familiar to us. The people, the work, the problems—all become parts of a "normalized" world to us, and we stop seeing many of their meanings. We settle on a few meanings that serve to help us get along with others, do our work with some degree of satisfaction, handle at least the small problems that routinely arise. But some of the problems persist, and these can become major headaches to us if we can't find any "normal" way to get through them, without changing things that seem not to be in our control. So, it can be very helpful to look at the same old parts of organization life in new ways, to ask kinds of questions that don't ordinarily occur to us. Such new slants on old issues are an important part of transformative "action research," a way of making critical inquiry a continuing tool of community life and work.

When thinking about organizational problems, we often tend to reduce them to single-cause explanations, when these problems are almost always more complex than that. So, ask yourself, are there other, possible "causes" of this problem? It's very common, for example, to hear someone describe a conflict in an organization as "just a matter of personalities." If you and your boss have problems, you may feel it's because of their personality: "They just don't know how to delegate." Or: "They're okay. We just have different personal styles." This way of thinking may miss some important questions to ask, such as about our organizational roles and responsibilities that also have their effects in producing or reducing "interpersonal" conflicts. Reducing conflicts to "personalities" may stop your thinking, and raising questions, about other things we might change, such as the roles and divisions of responsibilities in our group or organization. How do these roles create problems for the different people with their "personalities" who have to work within them?

Another common tendency that may unproductively stop our thinking is to reduce organizational problems to "bureaucracy." For example, it may be tempting to explain your difficulties with co-workers or supervisors because of their being in-grown, unimaginative rule-following bureaucrats. Even if people can often act that way, this way of thinking is too simple, and it just condemns them, assuming they can't change or won't. This labels them as stupid, and to blame for your troubles. Again, if we fail to ask ourselves lots of questions, we risk reducing things to such simple "formulas." *Instead, it's important that we try to ask a variety of different questions about organizational relationships, and if so, we may have better chances of getting new ideas about them, and also doing something to help.*

Here are some more challenges—about motives, goals, and money—and questions to ask, and there are many more that we can think of by getting in the habit of asking questions about things in our organizations and everyday life, that we may, at first, take for granted.

Motives

Every organization must call on people's motives to participate in its work, accept its services, supply it with money, or it would cease to exist. But the actual motives are quite complex. Some are explicit, such as willingness to work in return for pay. Others are implicit—you may like the work, find it a way to express yourself and to do something worthwhile in the world, even if the pay is inadequate. Your motives probably are multiple—you work for both pay and satisfaction or meaning. Your motives probably change over time; for example, your satisfaction may go down, and then your motive for working will change, also. Your motives may also depend on the situation or issue involved—when there is a chance to work with a group of people you care about, you'll want to do that. But you wouldn't want to do the same work for another group that you think doesn't deserve your efforts. These are a few examples of a complicated interplay of motives that are part of every person's life, and the lives of every group or organization.

Here are some questions to consider. What are my main motives for the work I do? How do they change? What makes them change, and what are the effects of their changing? How about the other people with whom I work? What do I know about their motives, and how do they affect the way the agency runs, how well it does its jobs, what kind of a place it is to work in? Is there some way to affect these things for the better?

Goals

Every "formal" organization, like a community agency, has explicit, stated goals—such as "providing low-cost health care to senior citizens," or "assisting low-income citizens to find employment." These are usually broad, flexible goal-statements that guide the agency, but leave lots of room for interpretation. So, different people and different groups within the organization typically may interpret the goals with different emphases, and these often conflict. One group wants more time spent on direct services; another wants more long-range planning, or research on the problems of the constituencies they serve. Some want to serve one group of constituents; some want to serve another. Over time, there may be a drift in how the organization acts out the pursuit of its formal goals, without anyone realizing it, but perhaps because people are responding to the crises and opportunities of the moment. As with motives, your own personal goals for the organization, and for yourself in working there, may be quite different from what the formal charter of the agency says. Your goals may change over time, as you learn about the place from personal experience, and are making your own judgments as to what it can accomplish or what is most important.

So, you could ask yourself: What are the "real" goals of my agency—if we look at the ways we spend our time and effort, as distinguished from what the charter says? What are the main arguments among us about how the goals should be interpreted? What people and groups have identifiable positions on issues like that? Whom do I agree with? How could we get together more on our interpretations? How well do my personal goals fit with those of this agency? How can I do what I feel is important here? How would I have to get the interpretation of our goals changed, to make my chances of fulfilling my own goals better?

Money

Money, and other resources that an agency needs to keep going, are important in every organization. Many of us find ourselves spending a lot of time, effort, and attention on getting funding, allocating it among things the agency does, figuring out how to pay salaries, and who can be kept on the payroll. We may find ourselves reducing all problems to money, the same way we may reduce problems to the "personalities" involved or to the "bureaucracy." We may feel that some people "are only here for the money," or that survival of the organization is so basic that other things must go by the boards. Such "purpose/survival conflicts" are realities in all organizations, so the point is not to ignore them, but to look for new ways of trying to deal with them creatively. Too often, it is assumed that survival must be dealt with "first," and then we can address the question of whether we are working toward our purposes. When opportunities for getting funds come along, it's easy to jump at them, even if they aren't for activities that are really going to support our organization's purposes. However, how much of our energy are we spending in this organization on what we think is important to do, and how much on whatever there is money to do? How much is the money the "'tail' that is wagging 'the dog'" (our program)? What are some things that we could drop doing, if we spent most of our time on what we consider our central purposes and personal commitments? How can we get money and resources to do the things that we really care about that would do the most for our community and to successfully pursue our purposes?

These are a few examples of ways that we can look at organizations, by asking questions that may not occur to us in the daily flow of work—but that importantly impact how we try cooperatively to meet the needs of own communities, and to act on our deeply felt commitments and values. Many other such questions can be asked, starting from how work is divided up, or about where we collaborate with each other and where we compete, or to ask what implicit values and norms govern our actions without our realizing it. If we get in the habit of asking such different questions, using our own, spontaneous observations of what is going on around us, we may find it is a big help in understanding how our organizations really operate. And that may help us to do something about it. Such question-asking is critical to transformative action-and-inquiry.

6

DATA-GATHERING AND SAMPLING

This chapter addresses the phase or step in the research process with which most people are somewhat familiar—getting information or gathering data. *It involves many important, seldom discussed considerations, and it also benefits from painstaking attention to detail. Yet it does not require precisely defined, standardized procedures outlined in most textbooks and guides to research. Although these procedures have their uses, in many cases, they may limit our taking a highly inquisitive, and necessarily, improvisational approach in seeking out information, or data, that, at first, we might not even realize are pertinent to our effort.*

Consequently, we will consider some thought-provoking notions about the nature of ideas and information, and how to become more conscious and intentional in our efforts. We will examine such specific techniques as interviewing methods, taking notes about our observations and insights, and getting information and food from thought in group discussions and from others in our everyday lives.

Related to "getting information," this chapter addresses methods of "sampling." There are many ways to do this, and the so-called, somewhat well-known "random sampling" is the least relevant strategy unless one is doing a carefully controlled laboratory-type experiment or large-scale survey. *I will discuss the value of "sampling for diversity" as a way to "broaden our experiences" to help us to obtain information relevant to our concerns from a variety of people and/or circumstances.*

This chapter goes into detail about the rationales and perspectives to keep in mind when seeking out data and information, including specific strategies and techniques of interviewing, observation, note-taking, and group discussion. The subsections are:

- Where do ideas and facts come from?
- Making it more conscious
- Sampling

- Broadening our experiences and information
- Note-taking to keep track of everyday observations and insights
- Interviewing issues, strategies, and considerations
- Eliciting ideas and information from others
- Analytical uses of group discussion.

Where do ideas and facts come from?

(Revised and updated from an earlier paper with Dr. Terry Lunsford.)
I suggest that we think of "information gathering" as something that is natural and that happens all the time, even though we are not usually conscious about it. Gathering and processing information, and using it in reaching conclusions, making decisions, and acting on them is not an isolated, specialized activity called "research," but the expression of basic human abilities, and something we all learn to do in the course of our everyday lives. We do it very rapidly, and usually without reflecting on what we are doing. For example, we gather and process data about the car coming toward us in the crosswalk, conclude that it may hit us, decide to hurry on across the street. These are the basic processes out of which research, and all that is called "science," have been abstracted and specialized, into a very powerful and complicated institution, with elaborate "methodologies."

Specializing and refining scientific methods has performed an important service, of course. Science, properly understood, does differ from our everyday information-gathering. Science tends to make somewhat more precise observations, to choose and focus on special problems, to separate those problems from each other and from the rest of life, from "action," for example. But these tendencies, as I have noted in Part I, all have their unfortunate, as well as their useful, functions. The bad effects have become worse, in many ways, as scientific methods have been refined and "clarified" so much, by specialists in "The Scientific Method," that they have been turned into a set of rigid, abstract rules, and formulas. These are designed to make us be very systematic and "rigorous" in all of our searches for knowledge—sometimes guiding us to give careful attention to certain details of inquiry, and other times, at the expense of curiosity, intellectual creativity, and holistic perceptiveness—all in the quest of the honored label of "scientific." Some of these rules are so narrow and dogmatic, and some people apply them so mechanically, that they become caricatures of what creative, working scientists actually do. Statistical methods, for example, have become so symbolic of "good" social science that they are used all the time in ways that have no meaning whatever—ways that violate the very conditions, which give them mathematical validity (more on this in Chapter 9).

I am emphasizing, instead, a conscious and intentional approach that builds on the aspects of research that flow most naturally out of the normal, everyday, broadly human activities, of which they are just a specialized, refined part. *We all observe, take in information, store it in memory, sort it into tentative categories, re-do these categories from time to time, come to conclusions, change our minds,* re-interpret the ideas and facts we are using—and go on about our business as we are doing these things. Thinking together about these activities—what is generally natural about them, and what is special to "science" is important if we are to engage in transformative action-and-inquiry.

If we think of a specific bit of "research" that we may engage in, we can ask: Where do we start? Where do we get the ideas that we pursue—about what to study, what questions to ask, and what might answers look when we meet them? This was discussed in the previous chapter and, this is an area much neglected by traditional research methods books. They seem mostly to start with a later step: "You want to study something? Just tell me what it is, and I'll show you how to study it, scientifically. But the problem of what to study, what the basic issues are, and so on, are your concern, not mine."

Fortunately, some people have given more attention to where our "starting places," themselves, come from. They have discussed these as being among the places where "science" touches and mingles most intimately with other parts of our lives and ourselves. Here are a couple of excerpts from well-known thinkers, who discuss similar issues from different viewpoints. They are presented here to stimulate and deepen our discussions and thoughts about "starting places," and about the interplay of research and the rest of life.

Michael Polanyi, in his book *The Tacit Dimension*, has explicitly emphasized the *"implicit"* roots of all knowledge. He starts with the basic insight that

> *we can know more than we can tell* ... He knows a person's face, and can recognize it among a thousand, indeed among a million. Yet we usually cannot tell how we recognize a face we know. So most of this knowledge cannot be put into words ... We recognize the moods of the human face, without being able to tell, except quite vaguely, by what signs we know it. (Polanyi, 1966, p. 4)

Polanyi continues on ...

> Indeed, any definition of a word denoting an external thing must ultimately rely on pointing at such a thing ... psychologists in 1958 exposed a person to a shock. Whenever he happened to utter associations to certain 'shock words.' Presently, the person learned to forestall the shock by avoiding the utterance of such associations, but, on questioning, it appeared that he did not know he was doing this. Here the subject got to know a practical operation, that is, a skill, but could not tell how he worked it ... Tacit knowing is seen to operate here on an internal action that we are quite incapable of controlling or even feeling in itself ... (Polanyi, 1966, p. 17).

Polanyi, a scientist-philosopher, emphasizes the personal, value-oriented character of the quest to know, to "discover" something that we have a "conviction" is there, but that we cannot fully describe. He sees this process of "commitment" and follow-up as happening whenever we focus on a "problem," to be solved. He argues that this means there is an inescapably *"personal"* element in all processes of discovery, which involve this purposive seeking after "hidden" truths. He therefore rejects much recent philosophy of science, which attempts to find general, "impersonal" criteria for the truth of a discovery or a conclusion (See Polanyi, 1966, p. 25). This perspective is reminiscent of our discussion of the inevitable role of emotions in science and inquiry, from the end of Chapter 3.

Quite a different approach, much more socially and externally oriented, is given to the origins of knowledge by the whole Marxist tradition of thought. Here are some illustrative ideas from a 1937 treatise, *On Practice*, written by one of the leaders of that tradition, Mao Tse-Tung:

> But how then does human knowledge arise from practice and in turn serve practice? This will become clear if we look at the process of development of knowledge.
>
> In the process of practice, man at first sees only the phenomenal side, the separate aspects, the external relations of things. For instance, some people from outside come to Yenan on a tour of observation. In the first day or two, they see its topography, streets, and houses; they meet many people, attend banquets, evening parties, and mass meetings, hear talk of various kinds and read various documents, all these being the phenomena, the separate aspects and the external relations of things. This is called the perceptual stage of cognition, namely, the state of sense perceptions and impressions. That is, these particular things in Yenan evoke sense perceptions and give rise in their brains to many impressions together with a rough sketch of the external relations among these impressions: this is the first stage of cognition. At this stage, man cannot as yet form concepts, which are deeper, or draw logical conclusions.
>
> As social practice continues, things that give rise to man's sense perceptions and impressions in the course of his practice are repeated many times; then a sudden change (leap) takes place in the brain in the process of cognition, and concepts are formed ... Whoever wants to know a thing has no way of doing so except by coming into contact with it, that is, by living (practicing) in its environment ... If you want to know a certain thing or a certain class of things directly, you must personally participate in the practical struggle to change reality, to change that thing or class of things, for only thus can you come into contact with them as phenomena; only through personal participation in the practical struggle to change reality can you uncover the essence of that thing or class of things and comprehend them ... (Tse-Tung, 1966, pp. 65–71)

Here, we can see that Mao is arguing for a close interplay of knowing and "practicing," or acting in relation to the things we are seeking to know. He says we must be in contact with things, to know them "directly," and that we have to change them in the process of learning about them. By implication, it seems, he would say that when we do have a lot of contact with things—patterns of events, social relationships, programs, ways people act, and so forth—we do learn a lot about them, although we may not be fully conscious of what we have learned.

These passages underscore the importance of learning from what we see, and practice, from our first-hand experience. Still, we can also learn from reading, hearing, thinking, and talking about the ideas of other people—first trying to understand them in their own terms, and then re-casting them for ourselves, to fit them into our own, personal frames of reference growing out of our own experiences.

The passages from Polanyi and Mao are quite different, and the differences are worth pondering. For example: Where would they agree, and where disagree? It is also worth asking, how do they know these things, which they assert so forcefully? Obviously, reading and discussing much more of their works would be useful in answering such questions. The point of reading them is not to persuade us to agree with either, or to accept them uncritically, but to illustrate some of the approaches that have been made to answering the question, "where do ideas and facts come from, anyway?"

This is especially important because, as we will discuss further in this book, ideas tend to give shape to what we consider the problems we want to do research on, and what we see as "data" relevant to solving those problems, and how we interpret the meanings of these data, once we have "gathered" them.

The main point here is to see and appreciate how much we bring to any research that we do. We aren't just starting out, with "open minds," to study "self-evident" problems, as if our only real task were to go around collecting the "real" facts and to see what they "tell" us. Instead, we come to any research project with many preconceptions, with outside pressures that shape what we treat as the issues of concern, and with very real social relationships into which our research must fit, and take into account—both the small-scale ones in our own organizations and community groups and the larger ones that run through the whole society.

Once we put aside simplistic versions of "fact gathering" and "rigor" as the only major issues in research, we can see that each of us also brings to it a lot of personal knowledge, and insights into the "thing" we want to study—at least, if it is within our environment, and we have some experience of it. Starting with something we know about gives us one leg up already, on the ladder of discovery. We are likely to have some pretty good guesses, with some information and some intuitions to back them up, about what we are going to "discover." That doesn't mean that we are already through with the process of inquiry, only that we probably have some *tentative* ideas. Next, we must get our ideas and facts together, to make clear sense of them, and to show others that we have good reasons for our conclusions. Still, we are well into the process, usually, by the time we "start" any action research project or defined inquiry in a formal or intentional sense.

Hopefully this discussion helps to build awareness of how we already know a lot, and of the ways in which what we already know can be used, very practically, when we are doing our own research for, and/or with others, in our communities, organizations, or professions. These insights hold not only for intentionally designed "research" but also for much of the thinking, concluding, and acting that we do throughout our daily lives.

Here are some things to consider. You might want to pick out some interesting area in which to do research, even if you later change your mind, and think about what you already know or think you know about it. Maybe you wish to study how well your agency or school is accomplishing things that you believe are important. Do you wish to better understand how and why the people in our neighborhood believe or think what they do about some proposed new policy? Do you want to understand in greater depth how and why some people overcome adversities when others seem unable to do so? Talk to people about the area of study and action you might be interested in pursuing more intentionally. You may want to consider some things that might be parts of the picture, but don't sound like parts of "the subject to be studied." Perhaps, if you are studying how well youth are learning to read in school, or do math, you may also decide to learn more about how much exercise they get? Or how "happy" are they? How happy are their teachers? How stressful are their lives? Many things may, directly or indirectly, be relevant, so which things are you going to spend some time trying to learn more about? These early thoughts in beginning inquiry are parts of that often-hidden "background" of ideas and facts that do so much to shape research as it unfolds.

Making it more conscious

(Revised and updated from a previous article with Dr. Terry Lunsford.)

Many everyday activities involve important aspects of research and inquiry, such as observation and talking with others. However, *research also involves more than those things we tend to do on an everyday basis.* Generally speaking, research requires adopting an "inquiring attitude" toward our everyday experiences and activities—becoming more conscious of what we observe, of how we interpret and evaluate our observations, of how we conceptualize patterns among a variety of observations and interpretations, and of how we ask questions and identify problems.

One useful tool for becoming more conscious about such things is note-taking. We often forget important details of significant observations and insights unless we make some notes for ourselves soon after the particular experience or thought. It is not necessary to take notes every day just for the sake of taking notes, but most of us probably have stimulating experiences and thoughts at least several times a week. It is a good idea to get in the habit of having a note pad handy to write down notes for oneself. Also, there is much to be said for the self-discipline of sitting down at least several times a week, even if for only ten minutes, to write down our most interesting thoughts from the last few days.

It is often useful to write about striking examples of compelling experiences, which illustrate some common problems or situations that we frequently encounter. There is no need to extensively document the obvious. However, it is especially important to look for unusual exceptions to the rule—to take notes about incidents which seem puzzling or which pose special or significant problems. If you have a special insight or idea, write it down and ask yourself, what experiences, observations, thoughts triggered this idea? You may wish to discuss some of these ideas, some of your particularly striking experiences, with co-workers or others whom you know. You can use your notes to bring out issues to stimulate these discussions.

The self-discipline of note-taking can be an important part of developing an "inquiring attitude." It's a way of making our ideas and experiences more conscious, so that we can reflect on them and discuss them with others. Another value of notes is that we can go back and look at them weeks, or even years, later, and learn much about our own processes of inquiry. We can look at the notes we take, and then think about how and why we thought about our experiences in the ways that we did. For example, to what do we pay attention? What kinds of observations and "facts" are we especially likely to notice? Are there some other kinds of "facts" which we may be overlooking? You might ask yourself, what kinds of information and observations do I, and my co-workers or close friends, give special attention to? Why do we emphasize these kinds of "facts" more than other kinds?

We can make check lists of things we wish to look for to build on the information or observations we have already noticed. Used in this way, we can be more attentive to matters of concern and more conscious of how we do research on an everyday basis. By contrast, if we uncritically adopt other people's check lists, or if we fall into a routine where we do not continue to critique and modify our own check lists, then we make ourselves less conscious about our action-and-inquiry. Then, we are using check lists as a "neat technique," as a "crutch," and we may have lost our inquiring attitude, and our action research is less likely to have transformative results. Check lists can remind us of some of the things we should be looking for, but we need not mechanically follow them as sacred formulas.

Just as it is helpful to think about how we make our observations, it can be helpful to think about how we formulate problems and ask questions. What kinds of questions do we consider important? And why? What kinds of questions are we asking? How do we know they are the "right" questions, or at least the "best" questions, "for now"? There are never any final answers to these questions but thinking about them is part of making ourselves more conscious about our everyday action research, part of that inquiring attitude.

It is also useful for us to reflect on the ways in which we interpret our observations. We almost always draw inferences from our observations. Consciously or unconsciously, intentionally, and unintentionally, we go beyond observations and arrive at conclusions. We may often be unaware of the observations, which have provided the database (or "experience base") for a specific inference or conclusion. In this way, "data-gathering" is always intertwined with "data analysis."

Some people might even argue that all observations are inferences—that all of us are looking at the world from some vantage point, which is the product of our values, conceptual frameworks, and concerns. That is, observations are derived partly from something outside themselves. At the same time, it might be argued that it is useful to make a distinction between basic observations, on the one hand, and the variety of inferences, which may represent different interpretations of a particular set of observations, on the other hand. To the extent that these interpretations are made with definite value implications in mind, these inferences can also be seen as "evaluations."

Further, we may ask ourselves, what patterns do we see among our observations? Such patterns can be starting points for our own theories. Still, it is quite likely that numerous patterns may be found among the same observations. So, we can ask, what observations do others make, of the same situation, or of similar situations? What are their interpretations and evaluations of their observations, and what patterns do they see? By trying to look at things from the perspectives of others, we can broaden our own perspective, and become aware of the similarities and differences among our various perspectives,

In research language, this consideration is basic to the issues of "validity" and "reliability," which will be discussed further in Chapter 7. A piece of research is said to be "reliable" to the extent that different researchers, similarly situated, will make the same observations, that is, come up with the same data. The research is said to be "valid" if we have good reason to be confident that our observations, inferences, and evaluations are reasonably accurate and meaningful reflections of whatever it is we are studying.

One good way to work toward validity is to try to look at things from the perspectives of others—to look at them from different angles—and perhaps, eventually, to discuss and compare the strengths and limitations of the various interpretations. A good way to work toward reliability is to set up "standardized" procedures, which will ensure that any two people will tend to make similar observations. One major issue and area of disagreement between social scientists is, should validity or reliability have a higher priority? What do you think? Is it possible to archive both? How? or Why not? These matters will be discussed in Chapter 7.

As an exercise, you might note some interesting and important observation that at you have made recently. Then, ask yourself, what inferences, and evaluations (if any), have I drawn from this observation? What was the process by which I made these inferences and evaluations? What other experiences and observations did I use? Did I consider more than one interpretation? Did I see many possible patterns? If so, why did I choose one as more valid than the others? How might I check out the reliability and/or validity of the method of inquiry I have used in this exercise?

In summary, an inquiring attitude is nurtured by our becoming more conscious of issues such as these that we have been discussing about the reliability and validity of our inquiry, and of both the distinctions and the interrelatedness of observations, inferences, and evaluations. Becoming more conscious of such issues can help us to get more out of our experiences to learn more from them in our action-and-inquiry.

It is through such critical reflection on our experiences that we can begin to develop our own concepts and theories. All too often concepts are formulated as concise but relatively vague statements that read like definitions out of a textbook. Instead, as discussed in Chapter 3, Blumer (1969) proposes, as an alternative, the "sensitizing concept" which employs a combination of a generalized statement or idea with specific, and varied illustrations and examples pertaining to the idea or the theory with several interrelated ideas. He goes on to discuss some of the considerations involved in developing sensitizing concepts—considerations which involve the kind of inquiring attitude I am discussing throughout this book. Blumer states that in research, the inquiring approach should be where

> One moves out from the concept to the concrete distinctiveness of the instances instead of embracing the instance in the abstract framework of the concept. This is a matter of filling out a new situation or of picking one's way in an unknown terrain. The concept sensitizes one to this task, providing clues and suggestions ... (Blumer, 1969, p. 149)
>
> It should be pointed out, also, that sensitizing concepts, even though they are grounded on sense instead of on explicit objective traits, can be formulated and communicated. This is done little by formal definition and certainly not by setting benchmarks. It is accomplished instead by exposition, which yields a meaningful picture, abetted by apt illustrations, which enable one to grasp the reference in terms of one's own experience. This is how we come to see meaning and sense in our concepts. Such exposition, it should be added, may be good or poor and by the same token it may be improved. (Blumer, 1969, pp. 150–151)
>
> If varied empirical instances are chosen for study, and if that study is careful, probing and imaginative, with an ever-alert eye on whether, or how far, the concept fits, full means are provided for the progressive refinement of sensitizing concepts ... (Blumer, 1969, p. 151)[1]

Blumer then concludes by noting that success in developing and refining sensitizing concepts "depends on patient, careful and imaginative life study, not on quick shortcuts or technical instruments. While its progress may be slow and tedious, it has the virtue of remaining in close touch with the natural social world" (Blumer, 1969, p. 152).

So, for example, if we are trying to study the concept, "trauma," we should not settle only on a 20-word definition, "trauma is ... etc." Neither should we merely define trauma as, "what is measured by one's score on the "Such-and-such" trauma index or scale. For example, as useful as the ACES (Adverse Early Childhood Experiences Scale) is to make rough estimations of people's previous traumas, at best, it is a rough, initial point of departure for future research (Kelly-Irving & Delpierre, 2019). Starting off with a tentative definition of 20 words, more or less, is an ok place to begin, as is a well-developed approximate, quantitative index, but the concept must be re-evaluated, further refined and fleshed out with a *variety of specific examples of different ways in which trauma can be manifest or shown.* As we learn more and more about the variety of forms that trauma can take, how it can happen, what it looks like with some people and yet differently with others, then, over time, we can improve upon our "sensitizing concept of trauma." We will be able to improve on our briefly stated definition *and* the understanding of the definition and *what it can mean* will be improved by having a richer, varied array of examples of trauma to reflect on.

Sampling

In doing research, the topic of "sampling" refers to the methods and judgments that one makes in deciding what "data" to seek and gather. That is, what is the relevant information we should look for to use in our inquiry—for example, what should we look to observe, and whom she would try to interview, and why?

By contrast, usually, people think of getting a "random sample," which is really based on one, very particular type of research, experimental research. With experimental research, the researcher chooses a group of people (e.g., willing college students), called the "subjects," and then decides to do an experiment on one subgroup and no experiment or intervention on the other group, called the "control group." The idea is to randomly assign some subjects to the experimental group, and some to the control group. The logic is that one wants the two groups to be "comparable," and it is believed that will be accomplished by randomly selecting the two groups, by what amounts to "drawing out of a hat" to see who will be put in which group. It does indeed accomplish that goal fairly well.

The other ways of approximating a random sample aren't really that random—for example, the Gallup Poll and other opinion polls try to estimate voter preferences among candidates. So, they try to obtain a "representative sample" of voters, since it's really not feasible to obtain a random sample of all California, or U.S., voters. If trying to project voter preferences in California, it wouldn't make any sense, for example, to only poll residents of Berkeley or any other single city or region, because it is well known that there are geographic differences in voter preferences. Instead of doing a random sample of all California voters, the pollsters will try to identify a proportional sample of different subgroups. So, they will try to poll a representative, proportional percentage from each geographic area, and within that from various subgroups (e.g., registered Republicans, Democrats and Independents, men and women, different age groups, and various ethnic groups). For example, researchers will take a random sample of people from each of the identified subgroups, such as for example, a random sample of the people living in each small census tract. This is called a "stratified random sample"—a random sample of each of the subgroups that make up the whole population being studied. However, in practice, it is not easy to actually interview or survey the people identified to be in a random sample of a large group. Many people will not be reached or will not wish to be surveyed or interviewed. So, the best researchers can do is to try to have a representative sample and try to get cooperation and surveys from as many people in that group as possible.

For the purposes of action research, the kinds of sampling that work for laboratory experiments and for projecting percentages for various surveys and polls are limited in their usefulness, especially if we are trying to develop new insights and new ideas/theories about people and society. As discussed in Part I, the medical anthropologists, Barney Glaser and Anselm Strauss wrote an important book, *The Discovery of Grounded Theory* (Glaser & Strauss, 1967). In that book, they suggested that even a case study of only one person, or one organization, or one setting or event, could be the *beginning* basis for developing a new theory. Once the initial theory is formulated, even if only based on a very tiny sample of people/organizations/events/circumstances, the next step, or challenge to the person(s) doing inquiry is to seek out some more to include in the study. That is, one adds to this very non-random sample, *in order to get information that will develop the new theory*. Over time, the added data or information from the newly sampled interviewees, or observed organizations or situations, will help to confirm the theory, refine or modify it, or lead to a fundamentally new formulation of a better, different theory.

Certainly, *this is in stark contrast to the popular image that "sampling" is done at the beginning of a study and then one sticks with that sample no matter what*. The conventional view is that to add to the sample as one continues with the inquiry would be to "bias" the research. Glaser and Strauss developed a method to continue to add to one's sample, as one gathers data, and analyzes that data. As researchers, we must *continually make decisions about what to look for next, what or who to sample for, as we get more information and as we do preliminary analyses of the data. They suggest that the more we learn about our topic of inquiry, the more we know how to sample, in order to test out and improve upon our initial ideas*. They go on to point out that: 1) sampling, 2) data-gathering, and 3) data analysis or not really sequential steps in a linear process of inquiry. Instead, these three "steps" in the research process should continue throughout the process of inquiry, and each "step" contributes to the other. Sampling—selecting "where" or "from whom" to get the data—contributes to data-gathering, and it also is informed by the analysis of data that one has gathered—each of the three steps or phases of inquiry coexists, and contributes to one another, in a kind of a continual feedback loop.

Consequently, it is important, to the extent possible, to do what I call "*diversified sampling*." That is, our understanding and ideas, and actions, will be more informed and more "valid" if we try to get information from the range of people involved in what we're studying, or from the range of organizations or circumstances relevant to our research questions or purposes. Most of us know only too well that some research is limited because information has been drawn from people in only one or two cultural groups, or from one kind of neighborhood, or that only certain kinds of organizations have been studied and not others.

Obviously, it is not always feasible to get great diversity in the people one interviewees, or the situations one observes. In these cases, it is important to think about and comment on how, in future research, others might improve on, and build on, our research by interviewing a greater variety of people, or by observing what goes on in a wider range of groups or situations. If one is concerned with how people function when confronted with a life-threatening illness, then it would be important, for example, to know about how people function who do have a strong support network, as well as by contrast, what's going on for those who don't have much of a support system at all. And, of course, for each topic, one can probably think of at least a few areas where getting "diversity" in the sample is quite important.

Another way to think about sampling for diversity, is to try to look for examples—situations, events, and people—that illustrate both the themes that one is starting to notice *as well as consciously and persistently to try to look for, find and learn about examples that illustrate the exceptions to the rule, the variations on the theme. Through this process, we can then begin to develop a more comprehensive theory which accounts for both the examples that "prove" the rule, as well as those that are the exceptions.* The resulting "new" theory is now better than the one we started with, better than the initial "general" theme(s). Even though the initial theory or themes might have been true, say 90% of the time, if we were to have done the standard statistical analysis, we can improve our understanding by "sampling for diversity" and by exerting conscious effort to learn about the exceptions. We are probing beneath the surface of the general theme, and most likely, we will learn more about the exceptions, while also benefiting from our understanding of the "general theme" or the more "typical scenarios." With this deepened understanding, we can formulate more effective immediate actions, and develop strategies of change, which are informed by the complexities and the nuances that are often missed by research which is satisfied with only knowing what goes on in the "majority of the cases."

Broadening our experiences and information

(Revised and updated from an earlier paper with Dr. Terry Lunsford.)
In previous sections of this chapter, we have spent a lot of time talking and thinking about the largely un-discussed issues of what we bring to research, including how we structure it (intentionally and unintentionally), how we make use of what we already know, how we prepare for deliberately "gathering data" about the social world around us. Then, we considered how sampling can contribute to research and action-inquiry, through a process where data-gathering, sampling, and data analysis, all interact and contribute to one another. In this section, we will focus more explicitly on some of the issues involved when we do data-gathering as such.

Getting information or "data" is an important research step because it focuses directly on our deliberate attempts to find out some things about "the world out there." This is what the scientific tradition has called "empiricism" and the more popular term today of "evidence-based," which is perhaps often used too narrowly. This means that we don't merely sit and ponder, or take stock of impressions we have already accumulated, but that we also try systematically to see and hear and smell and touch what is outside ourselves, in an area of concern that we want to know about in some detail.

Blumer's method of exploration

As discussed in Chapter 3, some people call the kind of research we are discussing "naturalistic." It seeks to see natural, human events, in their usual settings, as they occur with the least intervention from the person studying them, or from their "research instruments" such as questionnaires. One can study how a family lives, or how an organization maintains itself in a community, or how a program of social services operates. All of these settings will show recurring patterns of events, if they are observed over time—such as the ways a mother and her daughter "get along" or don't; how an organization's leaders act toward powerful outsiders; or what service agency staff treat as the needs to be met, and the services to be provided.

Wherever we see recurring patterns or themes, we can begin to describe them, and put them together with some ideas about why the patterns occur, or what consequences they are likely to have. Of course, when we start seeing patterns, we may also see occasional, startling departures from those patterns, which surprise us or catch our notice just because they violate some of our expectations. It's important to take note of such departures or variations on the themes, and to try figuring out what they mean, because they may enable us to see quite different patterns, which may finally be more important than the ones we saw at first.

Most textbook accounts of scientific research tend to emphasize the importance of having clear, systematic, and well-structured formulations of what you want to study, and set procedures for going about it before you start. As noted in Chapter 3, with the naturalistic approach, Herbert Blumer advocates that, in beginning research, especially, we should adopt a flexible strategy of *"exploration."* This doesn't mean sloppy or aimless observation. He means that the best, the most effective, way to learn about an area of social life is to immerse oneself in contact with it—personally, actively, with one's eyes and ears open, using all of one's abilities to see and understand what is going on. He means "a careful and honest probing, creative yet disciplined imagination, resourcefulness and flexibility in study, pondering over what one is finding, and a constant readiness to test and recast one's views and images ..." (Blumer, 1969, p. 40)

Exploration, Blumer tells us:

> is by definition a flexible procedure in which the (researcher) shifts from one to another line of inquiry, adopts new points of observation as his study progresses, moves in new directions previously not thought of, and changes his recognition of what are relevant data as he acquires more information and better understanding ... The focus is originally broad but becomes progressively sharpened as the inquiry proceeds. The purpose ... is to move toward a clearer understanding of how one's problem is to be posed, to learn what are the appropriate data, to develop ideas of what are significant lines of relation, and evolve one's conceptual tools in

the light of what one is learning about the area of life. (Blumer, 1969, pp. 40–41)

Blumer states that the process of exploration should seek out people who are especially knowledgeable of the circumstances being studied:

> One should (carefully seek people in the setting) who are acute observers and who are well-informed. One such person is worth a hundred others who are merely unobservant participants. A small number of such. individuals, brought together as a discussion and resource group, is more valuable many times over than any representative sample. Such a group, discussing collectively their sphere of life, and probing into it as they meet one another's disagreements, will do more to lift the veils covering the sphere of life than any other device that I know of. (Blumer, 1969, p. 41)

It is particularly important in exploration, Blumer says, for the researcher to be open to new lines of inquiry, as was Charles Darwin. One should

> be constantly alert to the need of testing and revising his images, beliefs, and conceptions of the area of life he is studying ... Darwin, who is acknowledged as one of the world's greatest naturalistic observers on record, has noted the ease with which observation becomes and remains imprisoned by images. He recommends two ways of helping to break out of such captivity. One is to ask oneself all kinds of questions about what he is studying, even seemingly ludicrous questions. [This] helps to sensitize the observer to different and new perspectives. The other is to record all observations that challenge one's working conceptions, as well as any observation that is odd and interesting, even though its relevance is not immediately clear; Darwin has indicated from his personal experience how readily such observations disappear from memory and that, when retained and subjected to reflection, they usually are the pivots for a fruitful redirection of one's perspectives ... (Blumer, 1969, pp. 41–42)

Many techniques may be used as part of this exploratory method ...

Some specific data-gathering techniques

Blumer's discussion of the uses of "sensitizing concepts" and his method of "exploration," along with my related comments about the importance of "sampling for diversity" as a way for us to "broaden our experiences," should inform and direct our data-gathering efforts. These perspectives can help guide us in looking for what data to collect, for what observations and information to look for, if we are to get a good view of the landscape of what we aim to study, both the "bigger picture," as well as the many, and highly varied details and not easily seen nuances of the landscape.

Using documents and records

There is a lot more to be found in the minutes, annual reports, memoranda, written policies, correspondence, and other records of organizations and community groups than most people realize. Lawyers and sociologists who spend the time to go into such records have shown that they often can reconstruct many issues and events that have happened in the organization, even without other people's help. Documents form a kind of "natural history" of a program, group, or organization, even if the people writing and filing them don't realize it, as they go on about their work-lives. Some of this history will be in artificial, formal language, and written from an official perspective, but other parts may not. Letters and memos, for example, can tell a reader a lot about the issues and directions with which the people in the organization have wrestled. Some groups put quite rich detail in their minutes, memos, and the like, which go beyond sanitized versions prepared for outsiders.

Documents can help you learn who an agency's important constituencies are, who the influential people inside the agency are, where the funding has come from, what the formal structure of the place is, and more. You will want to check out your understanding of these things, after looking at the documents, but they can be a good place to start. If your are studying your own organization, documents can help you learn what went on before you came, and how the organization has changed or remained the same.

Some people try deliberately to create an "organizational memory" of descriptive accounts and policy memos, for future reference. Mostly, you don't have to write detailed accounts, specifically for the "memory," but you can make the memory richer and more useful, to yourself and others, if you write occasional summaries of important events and patterns that you see, and which aren't getting talked about in official documents. This is especially valuable in a new organization or program, where things are just taking their first shape, and there aren't many rules, yet, and things are changing rapidly without anyone having much time to notice. As Blumer, and Darwin, note, it's very easy to forget these things. And, later on, when you want to look back and see where you have been, what has been accomplished, what mistakes you have made that you can learn from, you will find that the notes and memos you wrote, early on, are a gold mine of information that didn't seem particularly important at the time, but now are stuff of history. Even if you put it down in bits and pieces, a few notes, if they are legible, can remind you, later, of the "nub" of an issue or a series of events that were vital for the agency at the time.

Published research

A lot can be said about using research done by other people on the area you want to study. For our purposes, it is important not to be intimidated by an imagined need to "review the literature" exhaustively on something before you can proceed to do a hands-on study of it. Still, you may be able to learn some useful ideas or facts from what other people have published on your subject, and that is a good way to think about looking at some of the published research. Keep an open mind about this possibility and talk with others who may know about what has been written in your area of interest. However, a full literature search usually is a time-consuming thing, which tends to acquire a life of its own. It can too often divert, delay, and downright confuse you when your energies can be better spent, at first, in investigating and documenting the issues that interest you. Again, an excellent idea is to make notes for yourself, about any ideas, facts, or statistics, or ways of framing an issue, that you hear about, and which strike you as potentially helpful, which fit with your purposes and the educated guesses you are making. Use these as tools, as possible avenues, to follow up in your deliberate *"exploration"* and discard them or put them in as backup later, when you know more about how useless or useful they have turned out to be.

Participant observation

There are also many forms of this technique, which simply means gathering data by observing, and doing so for intentional research purposes, while at the same time being a participant, an actor, in the social setting that you are observing. Your participation can take many forms. You may be, at one extreme, defined completely as a "researcher," who is allowed to hang out and gather information in and around others while they do their regular work. If you are researching your own organization, group, or neighborhood, this may be difficult to carry off, since your other role(s) will get in the way, and confuse people when they see you wandering around, looking at things and taking mental or written notes. Especially if your usual role has some authority attached, you will probably need to help others understand what you are doing, and that you are not spying on them, to criticize them negatively. If you are in an unfamiliar setting, you will need to let others understand, in their own terms, who you are and what you are doing, in an ethically acceptable way. Usually, you will find that they soon go back to doing their work, without giving too much notice of you, so long as you don't represent some specific threat to them or to their work. However, there can be subtle adjustments in the ways that people act and work, when they know a "visitor" is around, observing, and you will want to be aware of that, in case the differences affect what you are studying.

In Part III, I will discuss some ethical considerations of research. For now, let's consider a few key ethical matters. First, it is critical that you respect the confidentiality and anonymity of those whom you observe. This means that in writing up your research results, or in discussing informally with others what you have observed, that you do not identify the names or identities of the people observed. This means that you may need to alter details about individuals that would indirectly "tip-off" others as to their identities. In most cases, you should keep the identity of the group or organization confidential, unless the organization has public or legal obligations and your observations are relevant to whether or not that organization is abiding by the law and its public responsibilities. Still, this is a gray area and gets into the more complicated laws and ethics around "whistle-blower" matters.

Secondly, if in the course of observing people, you do interventions that are beyond what you would do in your role as a "regular participant"—for example, by asking probing questions of others—this may raise ethical issues. Further, if you begin to ask probing questions of people who could be considered as members of an "at risk" group, there are added ethical issues involved and the likely need to have the individual read, understand and sign (or have their guardian or parent sign) a "consent form" to be interviewed, even if only informally. This is the case when asking probing questions, of children, of people who have experienced trauma and who might be "triggered" even by informal, innocent questioning, or others who might be psychologically or otherwise harmed by your questioning.

Sometimes, in doing participant observation, you may be simply a participant, in your own organization or a new setting. Meanwhile, you can make notes to yourself, as you go through your daily rounds, on issues that you want to describe or explain, in systematic ways, with data to back up your conclusions. You should, every now and then, sit down and record your observations and thoughts about them, while they are fresh. You should try to note the informal "hypotheses" that come to you, and to turn general impressions into questions or hypotheses—that is, into tentative conclusions that you want to check out further as you go along. Write down even your scattered thoughts, occasionally, if they feel relevant, because later they may turn out to have been the tip of an iceberg of an insight, just poking through your puzzlement and confusion. Ethical questions are pertinent here, also, and you will want to be able to talk openly with your co-workers about the fact that you are gathering data and analyzing it—if you have plans to do anything more than just think about what you are observing as a participant and inform yourself. Otherwise, you don't need to assume that ethics requires you to make such a big deal of this—that may confuse others more than inform them, and make them so self-conscious that they will hide or alter, in a well-meaning way, the very patterns that you want to study in their "natural" flow and setting. If, later, you decide you wish to use this information to discuss insights with others, or write up your findings, then you must go back and get permission from others, and you should be prepared that some may say "no" and that you will have to abide by their wishes.

Finally, there are many intermediate variations on the participant/observer dimension, which you may want to adopt as they are useful. All involve some advantages of letting you be in the setting while you are observing it—close to the action, able to rub up against it, to feel the feelings and intuit the relationships there. This is the great value of participant observing, as against laboratory artificiality, or the mechanical testing with some research "instrument," conceived and constructed outside the setting itself. All forms of participant observation also raise questions of bias, of your observation coloring the things observed, as well as the importance of your being aware that people always modify their behavior depending on their perceptions of the people with whom they are interacting. So, for example, a group of people who are different from you may act very welcoming of you despite the differences, and you may then decide that they are a "welcoming group." However, for example, if you are white, and they are white, they might not be act so welcoming if you were African American, even if they say to you that they are not prejudiced. Consequently, in making observations, we should keep in mind that not only are we affected by our views, assumptions and life experiences in what we are "able to notice and observe," but also that others will present themselves differently to us than they will to other people, because of our personality, race, age, gender, and much more. However, we will talk more about these matters in the Chapter 7 on Data Analysis.

As food for thought, you might want to think of participant-observer roles you have played, or are considering now, and note down some the advantages and problems they raise, and think of ways you might take those strengths and challenges into account as you do more participant observation in the future.

Interviewing individuals and groups

Blumer notes that group interviews with good informants can be quite useful. You will need to be aware, of course, that such group settings are public affairs, and that people will sometimes "play-act" or "make points" that they want you to hear, but which don't necessarily reflect the ways they act "naturally." Mostly, however, you won't want to take what anyone says or does, in your exploration, at face value. It may be an indicator of several things at once, including a clue to how that person thinks, how manipulative they are (or are trying to be), and who lines up where on issues that are important in the group's life at that point. For the most part, group interviews can be rich sources of information, especially in rapidly opening up your understanding of activities or relations among people, which you haven't had the time or opportunity to observe in person. The ways that people respond to one another's observations and ideas can be very revealing, if you watch for them, and can provide a way of cross-validating information.

Individual interviewing is another complex subject, with many, many variations, and will be discussed in greater detail later. Here, let's just note that an interview, as a source of information, can be anything from a casual conversation with a single question, asked in the course of observing or working with someone, to a semi-formal, sit-down talk about defined and pre-set issues, to a careful gathering of "responses" to each item in a structured questionnaire or interview "schedule." The main thing is to see that the observations, opinions, conclusions, assertions, values, and general perspectives of people living and working in any situation, such as a community organization, are all, potentially, "data." These data can have many meanings, depending on the contexts in which they are considered, but all may be useable as grist for the mill for your research. It's usually best to keep your conversations and formal interviews with others as comfortable, natural, and ethical as you can, without trying to manipulate them cleverly, so as to get at "hidden" meanings or facts. There is much to be learned from what people say, without doing that.

Questionnaires

This kind of written, carefully structured, research "instrument" is most frequently used in survey research, where one needs to gather large numbers of responses, about some definite questions or issues, from a large sample of many people. Typically, questionnaires are mailed out to many people, for reasons of cost, although they may be administered in person or on the phone, by interviewers, some of whom are highly trained for just this purpose, by large, opinion polling organizations. There are many things to be learned about the fine art of making a good questionnaire—such.as how to phrase your questions so they are clear, and so they are open only to the range of answers that you can deal with, in the analysis you expect to make of them. Still, questionnaires have been much over-used by social researchers, often to no particular advantage in getting useful information, and often to considerable trouble and irritation on the part of the respondents who have to fill out their neat, little boxes and categories.

In the next sections, we will pay attention to some specific techniques and details involved in using qualitative, participatory action research to gather data:

- note-taking to help to keep track of everyday observations and insights;
- interviewing strategies, issues, and considerations;
- eliciting ideas and information from others;
- analytic uses of group discussion.

Note-taking to keep track of everyday observations and insights

Previously, I discussed how note-taking can become a regular, not too time-consuming routine, that helps us to pay attention and remember some key observations and insights. By getting into the habit of taking notes, we can become more conscious and intentional about our processes of inquiry-and-action. In a more focused way, taking notes on your daily activities and projects can be an important way of collecting information on your group, neighborhood or community, or organization, and the activities that go on in those settings. These notes can also help you to keep track of your ideas and insights as you think about your work and your various community and/or professional involvements. You can do this on your own, and/or in collaboration with others. Through systematic discussions with others with whom you work, by pooling the ideas and information contained in everyone's notes, and by thinking about the implications of these ideas/information, it is possible to use these notes in 1) improving the effectiveness of your group's or organization's projects and activities, 2) writing reports for external funding agencies, 3) providing decision-makers, for example, Board members, with useful information which can help in setting agency directions and priorities.

Here are some tips on taking notes:

- Take notes on the reactions of students in your classroom, or clients and community people with whom you work, which suggest successes and problems involved with school or agency activities.
- Highlight crucial successes and problems. Don't take the time to write notes on every detail of your activities, but instead record those details that seem to be interesting or provide special insights.
- Keep track of your ideas, as well as your observations. Your thoughts and ideas about your work may sometimes be even more useful than your observations of "what happened," however, it is even better if you can connect your ideas and your observations. For example, did something you noticed one day stimulate you to think about a better way of doing an ongoing program or activity?
- After an important activity, write down just a sentence, or phrase, or two about what you feel was most worth noting. These brief notes can be used to jog your memory, later. At the end of the day, take a few minutes, say 10 minutes, for example, to go through these notes and fill in some more details and thoughts about them.
- Don't feel compelled to write about every activity, or even to write notes every day, but do try to get in the habit of writing notes on a regular basis, maybe at least three times a week, for 10 to 20 minutes each time.
- Take notes about a variety of different kinds of observations—sessions with clients, community program activities, staff meetings, and informal conversations with people. Teachers may write notes about not only classroom experiences, but what they see going on with their students on the playground, or in their conversations with parents.

Further, there is value in discussing notes with others. Co-workers can learn from each other by discussing with one another observations, ideas, problems, issues, and questions noted. These discussions may take place in formal staff meetings, or in informal conversations.

Here are some uses of the notes and the discussions of the notes:

- to catalogue specific types of successes and accomplishments;
- to catalogue problems to be worked on and issues/questions to be addressed;
- to compare examples of "success" and "failure" to better understand subtleties about when a particular activity works and when it doesn't; for example, why does an activity work in some situations or for some clients but not for others?
- to discuss ways of improving existing programs, to identify gaps in agency services or problems in classroom instruction, or to develop new practices or completely new programs;
- to discuss priority issues, not in the abstract, but in terms of specific experiences staff have had in trying to serve their communities or students;

- to keep track of what you have learned through your work, and therefore, to help you think about what you understand less well and need to learn more about.

Overall, taking notes, especially in collaboration with co-workers, can have some valuable organizational outcomes—not just from taking the notes, but also by thinking about the notes and discussing them together. Possible outcomes include:

- creation of a spirit of cooperation among staff in a shared effort to improve agency activities.
- intellectual stimulation for staff and mutual support/encouragement which can help to energize overworked staff people.
- developing a database for writing reports for funding agencies—a way of showing them you have done practical work and serious observation and careful thinking about your work. Notes based on your actual experience provide you with a way of giving them a tangible sense of what you are doing, and this is likely to convince them that you are serious and know what you are doing and what you are talking about.
- an internal evaluation of agency programs which can be used to make decisions on how the agency's programs and activities can be further developed, and about possible new directions.

Interviewing strategies, issues, and considerations

(Revised and updated from an earlier paper with Dr. Terry Lunsford.)
There are many types of interviews and ways of interviewing, inside and outside of formal research. Outside of research, interviews are conducted by journalists, medical professionals, counseling psychologists and therapists, and lawyers. There are specialists who consult with attorneys on how to interview prospective jurors, and many, many other kinds of interviewing. Even parents interview their children, when they ask, "what happened in school today?"—as do friends and partners, when they carry on a conversation. The purposes of these interviews vary considerably, as do the manners in which they are conducted. As a potentially useful learning exercise, you could as what you learn about "interviewing" in comparison with other interpersonal processes, such as "helping," or "flirting," or "negotiating." Think what things are different about them, but also what elements they have in common.

Interviewing for research purposes usually is taught as a series of technical issues or skills. Beyond the technical strategies, interpersonal finesse and sensitivity can be very important, such as for example, in establishing rapport or trust with the interviewee. Practicing interviewing is essential to learning it—by interviewing others, reflecting on the interviews, getting analyses and critiques from those who might observe you doing, or practicing, interviewing, and trying again. You can try role-playing or reviewing videos that are examples of interviews.

Here, I wish to introduce you to some of the many types of interviews, to some of the issues to keep in mind in interviewing, and to become more aware of the uses and limitations of interviewing. What you read here is not a substitute for further learning and practice, but rather a guide of some things to think about. I hope you will at least come to understand interviewing better as a part of a transformative approach to action research, and critical inquiry, in your everyday work and personal life.

With most conventional research, interviewing is usually treated as an effort to have neutral, standardized "administration" of a questionnaire form, with attempts to minimize interviewer "bias," and the "response bias" from the interviewee to present themselves in a way that they believe will make them look favorable or acceptable to the interviewer. However, it has also been found that sometimes interviewees will want to "rebel" against what they perceive as the "desired" response and say the opposite. This is referred to as "negative response bias."

Many questionnaires employ closed-ended questions where the answers are limited to a few choices, rather than "open-ended" questions which allow the interviewee to talk in greater detail about their thoughts, beliefs, behavior, feelings, and/or opinions or attitudes. The answers to open-ended question require much more of the researcher's efforts and thinking about how to analyze and "make sense out of" what has been said. Some people believe this introduces too much researcher "bias," but my perspective is that while this is a risk, the advantages are greater. These open-ended questions tend to elicit more in-depth information, which paints a richer and more accurate picture. The researcher is then less likely to misinterpret the meanings and significance to the interviewee, of what they are stating.

So, rather than trying to separate interviewing from everyday life, the transformative approach to action-and-inquiry sees that interviewing and research are both parts of our everyday life. As such, interviewing relies on capacities and impulses that we all have, and which we use spontaneously, naturally, all the time, with varying degrees of awareness and consistency. These capacities or skills include observing patterns in the world around us, forming hypotheses about their likely recurrence and their meanings, making further observations and checking these against our hypotheses revising our hypotheses, or making new ones, and then observing some more.

Natural curiosity about the world causes most of us to do these things, in spontaneous, flowing ways, much of the time. Paying attention to them, and seeing our observations as "data" for our tentative and constantly re-forming conclusions about the world, can be very useful in our community and professional work, and it can also make for a rich, interesting view of life in general. Interviewing involves all these activities and uses all of these capacities. Further, it uses them rapidly, with a lot of reliance on intuition, with many subtle "judgment calls" as to what is being said, and who is saying it. It uses evidence and hypotheses "developmentally," with newly learned information often leading to radically new hypotheses and shifts of attention.

Here is a worthwhile challenge to consider. *How can we make interviewing more "scientific," in the "best" ways of thinking about science and transformative action-and-inquiry,* without sacrificing interviewing's special virtues? These virtues include its speed, efficiency of information-gathering, natural spontaneity, focus on substance rather than the formalities. Also, it can be flexible and adaptable to one's changing purposes and questions of interest, and to each circumstance and interviewee.

There are many ways in which people engaged in community or professional work, teaching and/or leadership might use interviewing. Here are just a few examples, many of which provide valuable information that can then be incorporated into any research approach, including of course, efforts that are aimed at being evolving and eventually transformative:

- finding out what your constituents, learners or clients need;
- talking with co-workers about how to do your jobs better;
- hiring, evaluating, supervising, and sometimes firing employees, consultants, and volunteers for your program;
- advising or counseling (not necessarily therapeutically speaking) clients and friends, and sometimes including persuading, warning, threatening, and other interactions;
- seeking information, authorization, or other help from public officials;
- being interviewed, by people from the media, fund-sources, the neighborhood.

Let's now consider a few underplayed themes about:

- the types and sources of data from interviewing;
- the levels of meaning;
- thinking about interviewing strategies as scripts from which to improvise; and
- the relationships between the interviewer and the interviewee(s).

Types and sources of interview data

The explicit content of the response to an interview question is the most obvious type of data, but there may be other unasked and implicit meanings and messages that are conveyed. These include the tone of the person's voice and response, the jargon they use, or the way the interviewee addresses you. These things may tell you a lot about their personality, characteristics, feelings, and the roles they play in work and the rest of their lives. After listening awhile to what they actually say, and by also "reading between the lines," you may learn about their "internal frame of reference" or their special views of the world.

Levels of meaning in each interview

When people talk with each other, in interviews and in other ways in everyday life, there are often many levels and kinds of meaning that are present, and these are exchanged in every conversation and every interview. These meanings change and interact kaleidoscopically, and when we intentionally reflect on the emerging patterns, we often will see that there is much more to learn from than what immediately comes to our attention.

In interviews, there is always two way communication, with both parties giving and both getting information, considering it, putting it to use. The information the interviewee gets will affect their responses, and the future of their relationship with the interviewer. Indeed, the interviewer may consciously test out the *range of varied* feelings and views that the interviewee has on any topic. For instance, as noted above, in observing conversations among medical students, Howard Becker learned from many medical students that they were motivated to become doctors for materialistic and status reasons. To test the *strength and extent* of their feelings about this motivation, he asked them questions both in private and in public, to see how their responses might be different.

In most cases, it is really important if the interviewer can have a sincerely felt respect for the person they are interviewing, even if they may disagree on important matters, and convey a sincere eagerness to hear what they have to say. For example, in 1970, when doing research for my dissertation on a huge anti-war protest at Berkeley, I interviewed the heads of each ROTC department on campus. I anticipated that they might likely be in support of the war, and given that I was a young (even if somewhat clean cut) graduate student, I was careful to word questions in subtle ways that enabled them to express whatever different views they might hold. I didn't want them to feel compelled to "defend" the war effort or criticize protestors by my indicating that I had a position against which they needed to argue. In addition, I felt sincerely curious to learn about the various, and even unexpected, things they were thinking and feeling. I do believe that I successfully conveyed this sense to them, and this in turn made them quite willing to give me a lot more than standard, "pat" answers (Bilorusky, 1972; Peterson and Bilorusky, 1971).

Here are some further things to keep in mind about the layers of meanings and communications between interviewer and interviewee(s):

- Much of the information is exchanged non-verbally—by appearance, manner, body cues, intonations of voice, and implicit sequences of responses to each other.
- There is a constant interplay and calculation of what is being said with each person who is saying it. This has big consequences:
    a. Each person is constantly "guiding" the meanings communicated—and withheld—choosing words and intonations, using euphemisms as necessary, "presenting self" to the other.
    b. Simple misunderstandings of meanings are always probable between people of different cultural backgrounds, ethnicities, and social classes, and even job-statuses. These may be of minor significance, or they can raise issues of trust and mistrust, liking and disliking, evaluations of the other's character, politics, and the like.

96 Methods

    c. Attack and defense are always potentially involved, especially among relative strangers, with real or imagined insults to self and other being perceived from subtle cues.

    d. Subtle assertions of authority, and challenges to it, are frequent "harmo nics" to the things explicitly said. Most people have strong reactions and emotions to these issues.

    e. Most of these implicit dimensions of an interview are not readily discussed, or even admitted, by the participants until or unless they get to know each other well. Meanwhile, they are always there, and each party must guess what levels of meaning are involved at each moment—and what to do about it.

So, in subtle ways, as well as by the specific wording of the questions we ask, our interviews need to be tailored to our "audiences," to the people we are interviewing. Of course, the interviewees must be guided by our main purposes, and the research questions we want to learn more about. Note that although the interview questions may not necessarily re-state the research questions, and oftentimes shouldn't, we should design interview questions that are mindful of both our overarching research questions and also who our interviewees are.

Interviewing involves "script improvisation" rather than using a static set of verbal formulas

With a transformative approach to action research, interviews become a dynamic interplay of questions, answers, and judgments. So, in conducting interviews we encounter dilemmas, issues for which there are conflicting rules, and which involve split-second judgments or prudence in deciding what "rule" or principle to apply in the circumstances.

Quite importantly, how do we use some predesigned questions as "guides" for the interview, in effect as "scripts" from which we can "improvise"? How do we word our *tentative, and initial* formulation of the question, to be mindful of both our action research purposes and the people whom we will be interviewing? We will want the interviewees to understand the questions, and we will want to encourage them to say what they wish to say, without being overly influenced by our views. However, we may decide to ask people for their help—to let them know about the problem we are trying to solve and solicit their insights and expertise in helping us.

The questions we ask interviewees may or may not be our main "research questions." It is a strategic matter of whether, or when, we choose to ask directly our research questions in talking with an interviewee. We may do this indirectly at first, or likely only later in the interview, or in some cases, not at all. In any case, it is advisable to have some questions in mind rather than just "winging it," including possible "probes" to get additional, "deeper" information or to follow up to get more details. Also, we should be sensitive when it's not appropriate, either not useful or not respectful of a person's time or privacy, to not probe further.

Over time, after we begin a study, we may add interview questions that we hadn't thought of before, or that we decide are worded more skillfully and will elicit more revealing and relevant responses. We may decide that rewording one or more questions makes them clearer, or at least less misleading. Sometimes, we may realize that there is something relevant and important that we had so far simply not thought to ask.

This is very much like having informal conversations "in life." In the midst of talking with someone, we come up with questions on the spur of the moment, or maybe we decide to assert an idea or refer to our own related experience, in order to see what the other person has to say about that. We end up "thinking on our feet" as it were. This is just another example of the importance of improvising from scripts.

Over time, we will likely, and hopefully, learn some things we didn't anticipate, and when this happens, we should be prepared to update and revise our guiding questions! For most of the kinds of action research that I'm advocating, in order to learn about subtle dynamics and to generate new insights, it is not necessary to keep the same guiding questions throughout the entire action research project or effort. Indeed, it is desirable and important to be open to updating the guiding questions, to continue to delve into the emerging insights, the patterns, and the variations on the patterns.

Relationship between interviewer and interviewee(s)

From handling first impressions with the interviewee, to establishing and keeping rapport, there are many interpersonal nuances that are important to any successful interview. I don't presume to give straightforward "how to" answers to these matters, which involve interpersonal skills, as well as interviewing know-how. However, it may be useful to at least point out some things to keep in mind about your relationship as an interviewer with the interviewee.

Certainly, "rapport" is important, but so is detachment, so you can select meanings from the responses given, evaluate the worth and genuineness of what the interviewee has said, and guide them to staying relevant to your project's purposes. Sometimes these matters can conflict, or at least need to be balanced. Keeping track of time is important, so that the interview can be done within the time limit your interviewee agreed to, while still allowing you to cover all the topics and questions you hoped to learn about. Keeping the feeling of the interview natural rather than stilted or awkward is important, so that the interview can feel somewhat like a graceful conversation that has a spontaneous flow, even while guiding and directing the interviewee to address the questions in which you are interested. Further, one must continue to listen for the layers of meaning. For instance, how do you distinguish the words of a response from their "spirit" or meaning in context, and record the "right" one? How do you tell what is "relevant" in borderline cases? How do you keep track of the inferences you make from what you hear? Are there are other, possible inferences that you didn't make, but should consider?

Another important decision is whether to record the interview or to take notes or do both. There are advantages and disadvantages to each approach. In any either case, it is critical to keep the interviewee's responses confidential. An advantage of the recorded interview is that you don't have to take a lot of notes, and you can listen later to the recording, and even quote some of the especially important and well-stated comments. There are at least two disadvantages. First, sometimes people are more inhibited when they are being recorded, even though they have agreed to it. Second, listening to hours and hours of recording can be a huge time commitment, even with only a dozen or so interviews. It may be a worthwhile use of your time, but you should be prepared to do this, if you record the interview.

Another option is not to record, and to take extensive notes, and realizing that you can't, or shouldn't even try, to write down everything as though the interviewee were dictating to you. So, a disadvantage of this approach is that you can be so involved in note-taking that you aren't able to listen carefully to the nuances of what is implicit in what the interviewee is stating, and that you fail to stay on top of guiding the interview, by asking the best follow-up questions, changing the subject when necessary, and keeping track of the time.

Nevertheless, there are advantages to note-taking, and personally, I prefer to do a fair amount of note-taking without doing "too much." I take a lot of notes, but only occasionally try to write down quotes or near quotes to paraphrase very closely what the interviewee just said and use many of their words. If I don't overdo it, this keeps me mentally engaged in the interview without being too distracted by note-taking, and I've noticed that many interviewees appreciate my taking *some* notes, probably because it communicates to them that I value some of the things they are saying. Further, once the interview is over, I walk somewhere within two minutes of where I did the interview, sit down and spend 20 minutes or so writing down additional notes based on my recollections *immediately* after the interview. I end up with a lot of notes, without having been distracted in the interview—enough notes to have a good, well-rounded picture of what the interviewee said, including a few quotes or "near quotes." I have a lot of data to go through but not a lot of "extra" time listening to the tape recording "cold" after the interview is over. Those who want to be extremely thorough, and whose interviewees are comfortable with the interview being recorded, may want to do both—a fair amount of note-taking during the interview (but not overdoing it) along with listening to the recording after the interview. If you can commit the time, this would be, in my opinion, the best of both worlds.

Issues of power and ethics are always present in interviewing. For example:

- An interview is an asymmetrical, unequal relationship. One person is being asked to reveal themselves; the other is mostly not. Even aside from confidentiality issues, how much is it right to ask another person to tell of themselves? How much influence is it okay to exert?

- Motivations, needs, and desires to participate must be present on both sides, or the interview would cease. These may waver, and conflict, as the interview goes on. What does an interviewee "get" from participating? How much is it okay to influence their motives, needs and desires to get information that you "need"?
- Many people use interviews, as interviewers, and as interviewees, as opportunities for expressing themselves—their desires to be heard, to tell their feelings, to try out ideas on others, to make political points, to know about others' lives, to teach, to be "helpers" or "good" people. How these desires are shown, perceived, and manipulated are sources of both power and ethical choices.
- Even the simple issue of honesty is always involved in interviews, and not so simple after all. Shall I be completely candid with this person? How will it affect what they do and say? Is there a kind of honesty beyond complete candidness? How do I decide what to tell and not tell? Is there potential dishonesty in what I omit to say, as well as what I say, that is not completely true—as for example, when I played down without being out and out misleading, my own (strongly supportive) attitudes about students protesting the war, in order to gain rapport with heads of ROTC departments?

These are some subtleties that shape all actual interviewing processes, and they should be parts of any "technical" discussion of "how to do it," but usually are not. Becoming aware of them, and of the similarity between interviewing and other "natural" everyday processes, can help us to deal with them in the actual flow of our community and professional work and our personal lives.

Some common elements of interviewing, dilemmas and teaching interviewing

To summarize, interviewing may be defined broadly as "communication with a purpose." Interviews vary widely in purpose, setting, formality, importance, and methods. They are almost always a verbal exchange, plus much more. Non-verbal exchanges, many levels of meaning, very subtle processes go on. Interviewing always involves two-way interactions, information-giving, and perceiving on both sides. Sometimes there are fast, complex sequences of responses to each other.

Interviewing is an unequal relationship. One is usually asking, recording in some way, intending to use the information. The other is mostly giving, screening what to give, guessing what use the interviewer will make of it. Differences of culture, class, race, status, roles, power, gender, and other "social structures" are routinely involved, and they have consequences of which the participants' may or may not be aware.

Interviewing involves observing, interpreting, feeling, evaluating, inferring. Common sense knowledge is a crucial, "technical" tool used by the interviewer, no matter how "well-trained" they are, and quite importantly, the interviewer must "take the role of the other" in order to understand what the interviewee means by what they say and do.

Each interview has many implicit qualities and structures, like the beginning, middle and end of the interview. Interviews always exist in time, such as before/now/later, in physical settings, and in feeling tones such as liking/disliking. Interviews always involve unspoken judgments, no matter how open and candid the parties try to be. The interviewer and the interviewee always "know more than they can say." Prudence, judgment, insight, intuition, and a sense of "circumstances" are continually involved, and interviewers who are mindful are likely to elicit the most valid and valuable information and insights from interviewees.

Dilemmas in interviewing

Interviewers may often seek incompatible or conflicting goals, which create dilemmas for them, or require balancing acts that defy solution by simple rules or principles. Consider these challenges:

- Interviews require good rapport. However, avoidance of bias requires the interviewer to be detached to some degree from the feelings and concerns of the interviewee. Interviewees may perceive and resent faked good feelings.
- The interviewer must continually evaluate and guide the interviewee's behavior. At the same time, they must keep an appearance of natural, spontaneous participation in the process. This becomes a special problem when quick, efficient conduct of the interview is a demand, and time is short.
- Interviewers usually want, and need, more than short, formally correct answers to their questions. They want full, self-explanatory, accounts which provide some background and context. A challenge is, then, to fit these accounts into the interview time-schedule. Selecting what to leave out and what to put in requires many, sometimes unnoticed, judgment calls.
- Interviewers are usually asked to record the gist or meaning of what the interviewer says, not just the actual words. This involves interpretation, in light of the interviewer's beliefs and values and unspoken perceptions of the interviewee. These are not supposed to shape and color the data reported, but they always do.

Issues to be faced in teaching interviewing

The many considerations discussed above are relevant if you want to help others learn to do "good" interviewing, especially if you are leading a team of colleagues or community participants who are working with you in conducting an action research project. As you can see interviewing is complicated and involves a lot of choices and judgments. For example, how much attention should be paid to:

- broad issues of interpersonal perception and communication?
- competence in separating out observations, interpretations, feelings, criticisms, and conclusions?
- learning general rules to follow?

- learning specific techniques for narrowly defined situations?
- thinking through the interviewer's own approaches to typical situations?
- experiencing, feeling, and intuiting the process of being an interviewer?

So, as you can see there is *a lot* think about in interviewing—both about the content and process of interview, and with regards to the explicit and somewhat obvious, and the implicit and usually unnoticed and subtle. Next, I consider ways how inquiry can benefit from the knowledge, insights, and experiences of those with whom we work and interact every day, and with those to whom we can reach out.

Eliciting ideas and information from others

(Revised and updated from an earlier paper with Dr. Terry Lunsford.)
Over the years, in working with many different community people, community agency staff, and educators, I have learned that most of us know a great deal more than we realize. Frequently, we can turn our knowledge into useful "data" that can contribute to the improvement of our communities and organizations. Through the use of interviewing, techniques of note-taking and observation, and analytical discussion methods, we can sharpen and make fuller use of our natural abilities for observing, recording, understanding, and communicating about the world in which we live. Those of us working in community agencies or as educators working in either formal institutions or community settings can use such techniques to gather useable data in the course of our regular work, to put the fruits of careful observation and reflection into writing, and into practice in our daily activities. Some specific uses of these techniques might be:

- To use our own activities and experiences as important sources of data and knowledge.
- To learn from our successes as well as our failures, and from unusual experiences as well as from more typical and recurring events.
- To probe beneath the more obvious, surface facets of problems that concern us, in designing more effective strategies.
- To communicate what we know to co-workers, to others working on similar problems, and to funding agencies.

Further, as we elicit ideas and information from others, we can achieve other, important outcomes along the way:

- To enhance dialogue among grassroots community workers, community service professionals and community-involved educators, or innovative educators in schools and colleges.
- To mobilize people to act on community problems or needed innovations in organizations and schools, where such research activities as interviewing can themselves be part of the change efforts.

- To stimulate thinking and re-energize people.
- To facilitate networking among people from the same community or organization, from neighboring communities, and also from different professional backgrounds and areas of community problem-solving.
- To "hold a mirror up to ourselves" and to the problems with which we are involved, to get fresh insights and perspectives.

For example, the director of one community-based agency interviewed a number of co-workers as an initial step for program evaluation, and noted these positive side-effects: 1) It gave him an opportunity to think about what they are doing in a way that put value on their efforts. 2) He heard from less vocal staff. 3) It resulted in specific ideas and insights from staff that could contribute to program changes. 4) He became impressed with the depth of the staff's thinking, and he thinks they may also have been impressed with their own thinking when they heard themselves, since some good ideas came out that rarely come out in such an organized fashion. 5) People left the room, after the interviews, with better feelings about their work.

Meetings and strategies to elicit knowledge from ourselves and others rely on what we previously learned about 1) methods of note-taking and observation, and 2) interviewing strategies and issues. Next, we will discuss the special strategy of analytical group discussion methods to elicit knowledge.

Analytical uses of group discussion

(Revised and updated from an earlier paper with Dr. Terry Lunsford.)
Although it's not usually thought of in this way, group discussion can be used very effectively as a tool of analysis, of building new knowledge about a problem, of finding new ways of understanding issues. Community groups, educational organizations, and others that engage in analytical group discussion sometimes find they have a tool at their command that they hadn't realized could be so useful.

Group discussion helps in analysis, because, especially together, we all have much more knowledge about the places where we work and live than we usually realize. We know about the abilities of people, their typical ways of thinking, the things they have accomplished, the problems faced, and the things that have been tried and that have worked or failed. By discussing current problems, we face, we can bring out some of this existing knowledge and find its relevance to the present. During such discussion, oftentimes facts and ideas "just occur to us." Together we know more than any one of us knows, and it's fruitful for us to pool our knowledge and ideas. As we do so, someone, or several people, can take notes and pull our shared thoughts together. Indeed, we may end a group discussion with a new plan, or the factual basis for one, or a clarified problem that is easier to work with.

Such discussion can stimulate new thoughts, new insights, new slants on old issues. When done right, discussion is a relaxed but very engaged kind of work with others. It flows, and swirls, and jumps back and forth in very spontaneous, fresh ways that feel "natural," but it goes somewhere, something happens; there is progress and a product at the end to look back on and feel good about. There may be many kinds of products, such as a group agreement, new individual understandings, and a changed background of feeling within the group as a working unit, among others.

However, for group discussion to work well, some things are required. There isn't any "scientifically verified" version of how to do it just right, but there are some things that are known from experience to make big differences. Here are a few:

- Willing, comfortable participation. Discussion can be disappointing if a few people carry all the effort, or dominate the process, or if there is a feeling of being forced or bored or afraid of speaking up.
- Implicit ground rules that support and encourage openness and risk-taking by members of the group. "Brainstorming" can be very productive, for example, in creating new and un-thought-of approaches to old problems—but only if "silly" and "absurd" ideas are welcomed from anyone, and there is a rule against scorning or putting down anyone's contribution. Other forms of discussion may have different rules, but here all need to support diversity and openness in trying out ideas, at least as far as expressing them.
- Purposiveness. The opposite, but sometimes later on, complementary side of free-flowing participation is an unspoken agreement that contributions need to be somehow relevant to the issues under discussion. These unstated guidelines can change and become fuzzy at times but working with and around some such focus is quite different from having an unfocused casual conversation where free expression of anyone's random thoughts is acceptable. Helping others in the group feel okay about the process is important, but staying on the subject, or close to it, can be important during the process.
- Leadership. A skillful, comfortable leader, or leaders, can sometimes do a lot to help a group use discussion productively, such as by asking evocative questions, helping others to participate, and guiding the discussion's flow. It's best when everyone helps these things to happen, with one or two people taking leadership when and where it's needed.

This has been a long chapter, packed with details about data-gathering, and hopefully through all the details some themes are remembered, including especially:

- *the importance of continually modifying and improvising one's action research methods as we learn more throughout our inquiry;*
- *paying great attention to our personal responsibilities and experiences in conducting interviews, making observations (whether also as a participant or not), taking notes, reaching out to others for their input and participation;*
- *the importance of connecting generalizations from our insights with a variety of specific examples that illustrate the themes, as well as the variations and exceptions; and*

- *the continual interplay of the steps of phases of asking questions, gathering data, sampling for diversity and inclusiveness, and critically analyzing and making sense out of the data to figure out the main patterns and variations about which we have learned.*

The next chapter focuses especially on "data analysis," on:

- making sense of what we have learned from the "data";
- how we compare, critically evaluate, and judge the evidence we obtain; and
- examine the validity and reliability of our action research, along with the implications for action, and how to use action to then stimulate further inquiry.

End note

1 See also: "What's Wrong with Social Theory" where it is available online at: https://brocku.ca/MeadProject/Blumer/Blumer_1954.html

7
DATA ANALYSIS

In this chapter, I will discuss strategies and issues in analyzing and making sense of data. Many people focus on data-gathering without considering how labor-intensive data analysis can be. Oftentimes, researchers will enthusiastically gather a large body of data, but then once they have amassed the data, they don't know what to do with their data. In many ways, the hardest part of an action research project is to critically analyze the information (e.g., observations and interview responses) you have, and then to figure out how to interpret the entire body of evidence. This can be especially challenging since, with the most thorough research at least, there will be evidence which may at first seem to be contradictory or inconsistent. Wrestling with how to make sense of out seemingly contradictory pieces of information is important. Is some of the information more credible or meaningful? Is there a way to interpret the information, which although not obvious at first, is consistent with all, or almost all, of the information?

In this chapter, I will begin by examining the important concepts of "validity" and "reliability" that are commonly used to evaluate the quality and value of any research endeavor. Related to this, I will then ask that we evaluate any research project by examining the ways and extent to which the researcher(s) has/have been transparent about their research methods, and in particular, by looking to see if they have adequately communicated the details of their inquiry that led to their findings and conclusions.

Then, we will turn our attention to two important perspectives and ways of thinking about "data analysis"—making sense of our experiences and judging the evidence, and we will return again to considering how all this relates to "validity" and "reliability." The chapter will conclude by looking at how thought and analysis lead to action, and in turn how action can contribute to further thinking, inquiry, and analysis.

Seeking validity through transparency about one's research methods—the alternatives to "bias" vs. "objectivity"

"Validity" and "Reliability" are two technical terms that are often used to evaluate the quality of any research study. Because they are used often, and because the issues involved in deciding how to use the concepts in a meaningful way can be complex, the purpose of this section is to provide an introduction to the concepts and to discuss some of the issues involved.

The term "reliability" refers to the extent to which different researchers will get the same findings in each of their different studies on the same topic. Oftentimes, to achieve "reliability," research studies are designed using standardized procedures to increase the likelihood that any two researchers will come up with the same finding. I believe that it is very unfortunate that many researchers opt for the clarity and convenience of "reliability" at the expense of "validity." Before explaining why, we first need to look at, what is "validity"?

Although there are technical ways to define "validity," the concept of validity essentially refers to the extent to which a research result is meaningful and accurate in reflecting the complexities of whatever social reality is being studied. One good way of discussing issues involving the "validity" of a research study is to think about the strategies and challenges involved in weighing, sometimes contradictory, pieces of evidence. In action research, and in mainstream scientific research, the data gathered—the evidence—often seem to point to a very unclear and uncertain picture of what one is trying figure out. Consider a trial in a court of law. Opposing attorneys present the evidence that favor their particular points of view, and the jury must decide which body of evidence, *and* which interpretation of evidence seems to "make sense." Sometimes, the answer seems clear cut, to most people at least, but oftentimes, it is not.

"Reliability" is the extent to which most researchers, or in the above example, the jurors, arrive at the same conclusion. Or related to that, to what extent do the assessments made of the same "reality" or circumstance tend to be similar, even when done at different times and/or by different researchers. "Validity" is the extent to which the study, and its findings, are accurate depicting "reality." These may appear to be the same, but they are not. "Reliability" means agreement among studies—but what if most of the studies that agree with one another are "wrong"? Or what if they are "right" but they only paint a small, and not extremely meaningful, picture of reality.

Going back to our courtroom analogy, what if the "study" is designed to determine if the accused is guilty. And, what if in trying to decide if the accused was at the scene of the crime on a certain day, everyone, or at least most everyone who studies this question agrees that the evidence says the accused was at the scene of the crime? With regards to the inquiry into whether the accused was at the scene of the crime, there is then great reliability to that part of the investigation. Further, to the extent that the accused was likely at the scene of the crime, there is *some* validity to that finding. However, if the inquiry fails to address whether the accused actually committed the crime, the reliable "finding" is only somewhat meaningful, because the really important question about reality has not been answered. That is, is the accused guilty or not? Findings which are accurate, but which are not so meaningful because there are important details left out of the findings, can be said to be lacking in "validity." In this example, because the inquiry fails to address the important matter of whether the accused committed crime, it fails to do a well-rounded and meaningful job of portraying an important, critical detail about the reality being studied. In the social sciences, there are many studies which come up with a clear-cut, and even widely agreed upon, finding, but they may fail to address important dynamics and features of the reality with which one is concerned, and only investigate some of the more superficial, and obvious, features of that reality.

Researchers who take a more ambitious approach, who are trying to paint a well-rounded, thorough, and often relatively complicated picture, may raise more disagreements with one another and with other scholars. Their research may even be hard to "replicate," or to do again with the exact same results. However, sometimes these studies may accomplish much of value by moving us further in the direction of *beginning* to understand the complex reality being studied. If this is the case, such studies have some, significant "validity" (painting a good beginning, even if imperfect, picture of reality), even though they may be not so "reliable" (with researchers being more likely to debate and disagree about certain details of the complex findings).

Issues of, and concerns with, "validity" and "reliability" are also very much related to concerns about "bias" and "objectivity." Although researchers should make conscious and serious efforts to minimize how "bias" can lead to invalid conclusions, there is no such thing as research done completely "objectively" without researchers making human judgments during their inquiries. In Chapters 2 and 3, I discussed some insights from Kuhn's book, *The Structure of Scientific Revolutions* (Kuhn, 1970). Kuhn's research on the history of the practice of scientific inquiry revealed the central role of the judgments made by scientists, individually and as a group. In the section below on "judging the evidence," I attempt to show in tangible detail some of the subtle, and inevitably very human, processes and considerations in weighing and judging evidence (i.e., "information" or "data"). The process of judging evidence is not objectively done "at arms' length" by "unbiased" scientists, nor is it mechanical or formulaic. Instead, it is based on the judgments and perspectives of the individuals conducting the inquiry. So, matters of "subjectivity" vs. "objectivity" and "biased" vs. "non-biased" are not as simple and straightforward as many textbooks would suggest. Inevitably, reasonable, and open-minded people may judge evidence differently. In the section "Judging the evidence," I discuss some of these complexities, and the considerations involved in making conscientious efforts to evaluate the evidence more fully, more wisely, more critically, and insightfully. Even with such efforts and an open-minded approach, we can never be certain of our conclusions. Still, we may have greater confidence if some careful steps are taken, including, especially, reaching out to others for dialogue and collaboration, to obtain the benefit of their insights.

Collaborating with others increases transparency and benefits from others' perspectives. At its best, inquiry is not something done by a single person in isolation, but a continuing process that involves collaboration between two people, or even many people. It is not surprising that many, perhaps most, Nobel prizes in the sciences are given jointly to two or more people doing cutting-edge research in cooperation with one another. At times, "collaboration" involves competing scientists, each trying to get to a breakthrough before one another, but still taking advantage of, and building on, one another's insights. With this scenario, one scientist may gain superior recognition, but still all the scientists progress and learn more, as do the societies that benefit from their breakthroughs.

In fine-tuning and improving on our action research, getting additional evidence is always a good idea. *All evidence is "soft," to the extent that any information or data need to be verified by other, persuasive evidence.* A challenge is to piece together a variety of evidence to see to what extent they tend to confirm one another and/or raise further questions. In this book, I discuss some qualities of transformative action research, which if taken seriously, will at least increase the likelihood of one's action research being somewhat more valid, accurate, and meaningful, rather than less valid. *Some valuable qualities that may contribute to the validity of our action research are:*

- considering different situations and contexts, and the bigger picture;
- looking for specific examples to test out our insights;
- taking our own experiences and insights seriously, while also evaluating information from differing perspectives;
- looking beyond ourselves for information and insights from others, and especially;
- collaborating with others and getting the benefit of their analyses.

Given our concern with "messy," real world action research, our findings and insights will often evolve gradually over time, much like a detective trying to investigate a crime. Furthermore, the summary of what has been learned is often debatable. Our concluding perspective is in some ways like that of an attorney making their "summation" to the jury at the end of a trial, and only while presenting a very long and often complicated presentation of what may be seemingly conflicting pieces of evidence.

I suggest that in writing or telling others about our inquiry, we should honestly, unapologetically put ourselves in the "middle" of the picture of the entire story of the research process. Then, our readers/listeners can identify with our experiences and thought processes, and with how we struggled to make sense out of conflicting evidence and viewpoints, and then finally, arrived with our current conclusions and/or questions. Then, they will be well-informed when they evaluate how well they think we did, and why.

Unfortunately, all too often, those communicating about the "results" of their inquiry will try to take themselves "out of the picture." However, if we openly and straightforwardly present the story of the research, or action research, then our readers, or listeners, can better appreciate our process—what we began to think at first, then how we struggled to make sense out of conflicting evidence or points of view, and finally, how, after all was said and done, we ended up with the conclusions and/or questions that we now have. In effect, we should tell our readers the "story" of our involvement in the whole process of inquiry—what we did, including some of the key turning points during the process that changed and/or solidified our thinking. How did our data, and more importantly, our experience of gathering and thinking about the data, influence us to have new insights, more firmly rooted convictions, and/or uncertainties and new questions for further investigation? *I would add that by openly describing and detailing the key features of our process of inquiry, we are closer to being "objective" because we are honestly and transparently enabling others to evaluate the extent to which they agree with, disagree with, and/or question our process and our conclusions. Further, we are actively inviting them to be, engaged in this continuing inquiry with us.*

I learned much about this approach from Howard Becker's wonderful article on "Problems of Inference and Proof in Participant Observation" in which he articulates the importance of being transparent about our evolving research, our activities, and our resulting insights, by "telling the story" of our inquiry. Becker suggests that sociologists can write and give "proof" of their conclusions by "a description of the natural history of our conclusions, presenting the evidence as it came to the attention of the observer during successive stages of his conceptualization of the problem" (Becker, 1958, p. 660).

Consequently, an important part of the research process, of scientific inquiry, is communicating what we know to others—not just "what" we know, or think, or believe that we know, but also *how* we came to those conclusions or ideas. The better we inform others about how we came to our conclusions, the more successful we are in being *transparent* about our methods of inquiry. Public transparency is one of the cornerstones of good science and enables us to assess the validity of any research. *We cannot be completely "objective," but we can try to be systematic, critically minded, highly inquisitive and open-minded, and transparent. Trying to adopt and practice these qualities, including transparency, is better than whether we use numbers and statistics, more important than whether we adopt a particular research design, or any single research procedure. If we are transparent, then others will be able to evaluate our research, or action research, and decide how confident that they wish to be in our findings. They can decide in what ways our findings seem to be "valid" and in what ways, limited.*

Making sense out of experiences

(Revised and updated from an earlier paper with Dr. Terry Lunsford.)

We are now in the realm of "data analysis." It is one thing for us to gather data, and to use our own experiences as "data," but it involves a further step to begin to examine that data. We are now going to give attention to how we can analyze our or make sense out of our experiences. Just as the discussion on "mining our experiences" involved considerations beyond conventional data-gathering, so do the notions of "making sense out of experiences" and "making judgments" or "judging the evidence" lead us to issues and methods which go beyond what some see as "data analysis."

The choice of the term "making judgments" is revealing. In making judgments we may sometimes be thinking about taking action, for in deciding what to do, we make judgments. Sometimes, we make judgments almost impulsively, or perhaps intuitively, but other times we make judgments after a lengthy process of reflection. So, how can we make our processes of making judgments more "systematic"? How can we be more thorough in paying attention to the "facts"? How can we decide which facts are most relevant to the judgment process, and in the circumstances with which we are concerned? How can we improve the thinking we bring to such a process? The word "judgments" suggests that our values and purposes are very much part of this process, and of course, they are.

Inevitably, we do make judgments, and we are continually involved in making sense out of our experiences. There is much that is valuable and creative in our "natural" involvement in these processes; that is why many people place such a high value on their natural insights, following their instincts, acting on their intuition, on "doing what seems right." At the same time, *we may fruitfully ask ourselves the question, can we do particular things, which may lead us to deeper insights and to more creative alternatives for action as we go about the everyday work of making sense out of our experiences? Are there some considerations and methods of inquiry, which can help us to do more than merely to act out of "common sense"?*

Increasingly, conventional research downplays the role of critical and creative thinking and employs artificial intelligence or uses statistical models. Many research projects devote vast amounts of time and energy to data-gathering, and then at the end of the project the masses of data accumulated are poured into a computer with the hope that one of several intricate computer programs will somehow make sense out of the data. Nevertheless, in important ways, our purposes and values, as well as our ideas, hunches and past experiences, provide frameworks for data analysis, in ways that are similar to, but quite more complex than, a computer program that tells the computer how to analyze a body of data.

This is especially the sort of thinking that Hugh and Stuart Dreyfus (Dreyfus & Dreyfus, 1985) discuss as what highly experienced people do at the more advanced levels of expert knowledge. *With some degree of experience and practice, as well as deep and expansive thinking, we all can engage in analyses that are quite complex.* Our efforts to make sense out of data cannot be reduced to a computer program unless we intentionally engage in special, and highly self-disciplined efforts to restrict and simplify our thinking. Ironically, some social researchers do exactly this in efforts to make their analysis of the data "objective." Our own natural frameworks for making sense out of data/experience are not necessarily any more or less "subjective" than a particular computer program, which after all is a codified process of thinking created by human minds for consumption and use by computers. Potentially, at least, the concerns, questions, and methods which guide our analysis of data can be more in touch with the realities we are trying to understand and/or act on, or make judgments about, than any standardized, or computerized, process of analysis.

What are some things that we can keep in mind to make "better" sense out of experiences? Blumer suggests that we consider a process he calls "inspection" (Blumer, 1969). We should inspect our data by asking different questions of the data. We should look at the data from different angles, maybe even ask a variety of others to look at the data and share with us what sense they get from the data. By looking at the data from different angles, we may make various comparisons between "slices of the data." That is, we may group the "pieces" of data in different ways, compare the pieces for similarities and differences, and see what kinds of ideas come to us as we pattern our data or experiences in different ways. In our mind's eye, we may arrange and rearrange the facts in different ways, to ask questions of the facts. Each pattern may tell a slightly different, or maybe occasionally even a profoundly different, story.

For example, suppose our concern is, "why do people get high blood pressure?" We may rephrase this question and come up with different questions to ask of the data. Here are two examples. Why do individuals get high blood pressure in our society? Why does high blood pressure exist in the society? Both questions are relevant, but each question suggests a different approach to making sense out of data. The first question might very well lead us to a comparison of case records about different individuals, individuals who have high blood pressure and individuals who don't. We might even make comparisons between individuals of the same age, race, or sex. Alternatively, we might look at those individuals who have the characteristics commonly associated with high blood pressure, and the compare those who have high blood pressure with those who don't.

The second question might lead us to group data in somewhat different ways. We might compare individuals from different walks of life in the society—wealthy people and poor people, employed people and unemployed people, people living in neighborhoods with a low incidence of high blood pressure to people in areas where high blood pressure is more common. We might collect additional data—to get more information on different societies and different communities rather than focusing only on individual cases.

This leads us to another point. After analyzing some data, after trying to make sense out of some experiences or body of data, we may then gain added insight into what new data to collect, in order to broaden our experiences and our knowledge, in order to pursue the questions we consider important. Here we see research as a continuing process. There is an ongoing interplay between collection of data—that is, taking action and broadening our experiences, on the one hand and analyzing data, and making sense out of experiences, on the other hand. Each one feeds into the other and informs the other.

Going back to our example, we might also note that the questions we ask of the data are likely to follow from and/or lead to consideration of certain courses of action. For example, the first question might closely relate to the action-oriented issue, what can I do to meet the health needs of individuals in the community?

Whereas the second example might relate more directly to, what community-oriented actions would improve conditions which affect the health of people in the community? These two sets of questions are not incompatible, but do suggest different emphases in our concerns, purposes, and the general direction of our inquiry.

So, it is often thought-provoking to try to ask many different questions, and to pursue different lines of inquiry when looking at any body of data or number of experiences. It is important that we ask questions, which are relevant to our purposes, values, and concerns; unfortunately, this rather basic principle of inquiry is often ignored by standardized research procedures. At the same time, as noted above, it may be illuminating to force ourselves to look at data in new ways, to get other people to help us by sharing their impressions. This may help us to avoid becoming bogged down in narrowly defined concerns, in misguided or ill-informed purposes, and generally in unexamined ways of making sense out of the facts and experiences we encounter.

All this suggests that *we need to thoughtfully immerse ourselves in the data.* We should feel free to play around with the data, trying out hunches, making educated guesses, putting the pieces of data together in different ways, trying out different explanations and interpretations of the data, and then making some judgments about or further investigations into the accuracy and relevance of these various different explanations. This creatively reflective process should not merely be a haphazard adventure into speculation, either. We can look for trends and patterns of facts, which support different judgments (e.g., theories or courses of action), and then we can look for "exceptions" and for data that contradict those themes. We should ask questions about these exceptions to the rule. What sense can we make out of these disturbing or puzzling pieces of information? Can we think of a new pattern, which makes sense out of the initial pattern, and also the puzzling exceptions? If so, we are very probably making progress—that is, we are very probably making "more sense" out of the data.

We should try to generate an alternative scenario—that is, try to conceptualize different possible patterns of facts, or possible future courses of action—and then look at our data in light of these alternatives. Which alternatives seem to be most consistent with our experiences, or with the facts, as we understand them? We must be open to the new, unusual and unexpected, and we should also try to consciously become attuned to ways of making our inquiry more systematic and probing. As Howard Becker suggests,

> The best evidence may be that gathered in the most unthinking fashion, when the observer has simply recorded the item although it has no place in the system of concepts and hypotheses he is working with at the time, for there might be less bias produced by the wish to substantiate or repudiate a particular idea. On the other hand, a well-formulated hypothesis makes possible a deliberate search for negative cases ... (Becker, 1958)

In other words, there are two, seemingly opposite aims, which I'll refer to as "verification" and "curiosity," in our efforts to make sense of experiences, of the data, and both are important. Oftentimes, however, researchers place a great emphasis on "verification" at the expense of "curiosity." "Curiosity" aims at generating new ideas, new insights, new interpretations, and generally with discerning different patterns within the data, that is, coming up with different concepts or formulations of the data. The verification emphasis focuses on critically examining the accuracy and relevance of a particular interpretation of the data, and substantiating or refuting the validity and value of that interpretation.

With transformative action research, there is most often a continuing interplay between these two aspects—curiosity and verification, and oftentimes continued curiosity and further verification. Curiosity and/or verification can lead us to action, further experience, and in the process more data, new ideas, and the cycle of curiosity-action-verification continues as transformative action-and-inquiry. It should be added that the cycle can begin with action, which will then engage us in exercising curiosity and engaging in verification. These three different emphases of action, curiosity, and verification can evolve in any combination of sequences, and sometimes they may even be going on at the same time.

To illustrate how the interpretations and judgments which follow from any particular body of facts depend on one's purposes and concerns let's consider a 40-year-old-story about action research pursued by Michael Bennett, a 37-year-old journeyman pipefitter at the General Motors Fisher Body plant on Coldwater Road in Flint, Michigan (Howard, 1981):

> In 1977, Bennett became suspicious about what seemed to be an unusually high number of his fellow workers who were suffering, and dying, from cancer. So when he was elected president of the United Auto Workers local 326 in 1978, Bennett decided to do something about it. Over the next two years, Bennett documented rates of cancer among Coldwater Road workers two and three times the normal rate in a comparable population, setting into motion a major cancer alert at the GM-Fisher Body plant. [Note how Bennett's research began with an inquiry phase that was very much part of his everyday experience and then he moved into a phase which, was more oriented to verification when he documented rates of incidence of cancer.] According to the Detroit News, "Bennett's work has drawn attention to the health hazards that exist in the automotive industry and paved the way for future investigations …"
>
> This then lead to further research by United Auto Workers, and this research emphasized inquiry into the possible causes of cancer; this has led to new hypotheses at a deeper level of insight—this time not just about the presence of cancer-causing work conditions, but now about what it is in those conditions which is cancer-causing. Presently, there is a pattern of evidence pointing toward exposure to a family of chemicals, known as PAHs. Consider these comments made by UAW epidemiologist:
>
>> We have serious concerns about PAHs in the industry, concerns backed up by a substantial amount of documentation. But with respect to this particular

plant, we don't have the data to point the finger at PAHs as opposed to other chemicals. (Howard, 1981)

This *In These Times* article goes on to describe the difference in interpretation and judgment between union and corporate officials in light of this data:

> This lingering uncertainty has shaped the negotiations between the UAW and General Motors about what to do at Coldwater Road and about occupational cancer in general. The UAW has adopted a preventive approach that considers any indication, however preliminary, of high cancer rates as grounds for "presumptive action." While the conditions at Coldwater Road have improved considerably over the last 10 years, union experts say there are still changes to be made. Moreover, new hazards are probably being introduced along with the toxic substances used in urethane plastics production. "We don't really know what the risks are with these new materials …"
>
> For that reason, the union is negotiating with GM for action in three areas: increased medical surveillance of the Coldwater Road workforce, including worker education programs about occupational cancer; further epidemiological research; and engineering controls to protect workers from potential hazards …
>
> In contrast to the union's preventive approach, however, General Motors has emphasized the cautious search for scientific certainty—hard proof linking high cancer rates to specific substances in the workplace … "The only thing we know is that it appears there is an elevated incidence of cancer of the lung," says Dr. Robert Wiencek, director of occupational safety and health for General Motors. "Is it due to workplace exposures? Sure, it could be. But it could also be something else. We really don't know enough about the problem to say. The indications are there; there is no doubt about that. But we need more time." (Howard, 1981)

In this story of competing studies, we have the same data, but different interpretations, different judgments, with different implications for action and different suggested directions for further research. Rather obviously, the studies are being conducted by people with different interests, and concerns. Still, we might ask, How could we make use of these two different perspectives if we were going to be involved in this situation—in doing research, in taking action—in making judgments and making sense out of data? For example, could it be that there is some "truth" in both perspectives? Stated differently, could we use both perspectives, to give us a deeper insight into the facts being considered? If so, how? One explanation that accounts for both conclusions, of course, is that the emphasis on "conclusive" verification serves General Motor's interests, whereas workers understandably want to minimize their risks, and don't want to wait for conclusive verification in order to protect their well-being, "just in case." Nevertheless, there may be additional ways of taking into account both perspectives, at least to some extent.

Applying this lesson, each of us might think of two different interpretations of experiences/data relevant to our own professional or community work, and then reflect on how to make sense out of things by using both perspectives, somewhat at least. *Let's see if we can consider the value of a "both/and" way of looking at things, rather than only "either/or."*

Here's an exercise. Write down some notes about some significant, related experiences and/or other data relevant to your organization, community, professional group, or any important situation you wish to examine. Try to look at these facts in a way which will help you to see the situation, or your organization or community, as being both unique and similar to some other situations, agencies, or groups. This can be helpful because we sometimes get so wrapped up in our own experiences that we think that our experiences are completely subjective or distinctive to our particular circumstances or us. We sometimes lose sight of the fact that our situation is most likely also a microcosm or example of a larger trend.

To take another example, if we are studying an educational process, we might tend to formulate an "either/or" type of question such as, is this educational process liberating or oppressive? In doing so, we might overlook the important, and perhaps likely, possibility that the educational process being examined is both liberating and oppressive. Perhaps in some ways, it is enlightening, it encourages initiative, helps people to think for themselves, to learn from each other, and helps people to be aware of the impact of systemic societal forces. Nevertheless, it might at the same time, in some ways limit people's imagination, perpetuate certain kinds of injustices by legitimating special access to resources for an select, elite group of people, or encourage us merely to "react" against things that remind of us of conventional education, even when they could be beneficial. This kind of logic and inquiry—emphasizing "both/and"—is called *dialectical logic*. It emphasizes a critical analysis which avoids neat and simple interpretations—it assumes that the world is likely to be a messy and complicated place where the insights from our experiences may simultaneously and accurately lead us in two seemingly different directions.

In using a "both/and" perspective, our efforts in "making sense out of experiences" becomes more interesting, less frustrating, and more insightful and meaningful. This doesn't mean that both perspectives have equal weight or validity, but that often, each perspective can contribute some things of value to our transformative approach to action-and-inquiry.

Judging the evidence

(Revised and updated from an earlier paper with Dr. Terry Lunsford.)

Now, I'll shift to several specific questions that come up as we assess and evaluate data, the conclusions toward which we are moving, and the ways the two processes of "making sense" and "judging" go together.

Facts, conclusions, and arguments in action research

When look at facts as "evidence," and judge them, it may seem obvious that we are already considering facts in relation to something else—a conclusion, assertion, statement, or "finding," which we think the "facts" tend to support, or to establish as true. That is, "evidence" is supportive proof for or against something, and that something usually is a conclusion that we are arguing, or at least tentatively suggest to ourselves and others as true.

This is important to discuss, because we need to understand that the assertion or conclusion that we are aiming toward will help to notice as relevant what "facts" that we should select and record. If our tentative conclusion, for example, is that a program is meeting specific, planned needs of its constituents, then we will look for "facts" that support or deny that conclusion, without perhaps realizing that there are always many other facts around, which we may want to notice, and make use of, as well. That is why starting with a richly descriptive account of "what is going on," based on a broadly cast net for "facts" is usually important for productive action research. This is what I meant in the previous chapter by the value of "broadening our experiences," of "diversified sampling," and Blumer's concept of exploration. By contrast, starting out immediately with a narrow hypothesis to be tested is a common error of people who have been schooled too rigorously in conventional versions of research method.

I have also previously suggested that using your own, intuitive hunches, and "everyday facts" that you already have observed, is very much advised in action research. However, it does make sense, after you have begun getting your descriptive and intuitive accounts well-stated, to start formulating and listing the kinds of conclusions you expect you might reach, and to line up the facts that have something to do with them. There is no reason why you shouldn't begin by pointing generally toward the conclusions you want or expect to reach. In other words, just because you want to believe something is true (such as, "We are doing the job!") doesn't mean that you can't research that question—or that you should pretend to be neutral about it. The better way is to be clear about your hoped for or anticipated conclusions, is to use them in the form of working hypotheses; that is, as tentative conclusions, which are to be tested by research. Then you can continue, using your descriptive account as a running start, to "build the case" for and against your hypotheses, and open them up to others for their comment and criticism. And, ideally, you can also inquire with curiosity to generate some other hypotheses.

It may help to recall that all scientific conclusions are tentative. This is true, not just for hypotheses, but also for the findings of elaborate studies, and especially for the "conclusions" of such studies. All are true only to a degree, depending on the quality of the evidence presented for them, the sense and coherence they make for us, the aptness of the way the conclusions are stated, the ways they test out in practice, and the extent to which they seem to be meaningful or important. This doesn't mean that "there is no science" or "verified truth," but that all "verification" is partial, based on incomplete and imperfect evidence. So, it isn't necessary to pretend or try for an imaginary, "scientific detachment." It does make sense to get clear for yourself what you are investigating, what your purposes are, what you "hope" is true, and what kinds of skepticism and criticism you are likely to face when you "go public" with your findings.

It's not that "bias," and "wishing-it-were-true," don't make any difference; they do. For example, if you are committed to pushing some dogmatic conclusion, as lawyers have to be when committed to their clients' interests, you are likely to overdraw the evidence for that cause, and to slight or distort the evidence against it. That is one reason why the scientific traditions have emphasized transparency, while also looking carefully at the evidence against your hypothesis, as well as that which supports it. It's like starting the dialogue with your colleagues and critics, beforehand, by having that dialogue with yourself. It involves asking yourself questions such as, what "makes" me think that we're achieving our goals? What kinds of things make me doubt it? How can I find out more about both of those? If you layout your conclusions, the way you hope they will turn out, you can then write down the pros and cons that you have observed or gathered, and tote them up, to see where you come out on the first trial run in analyzing your data. You may have to jiggle, and re-word, and adjust the hypotheses and the evidence a few times, but pretty soon you'll have a meaningful, internally relevant picture of what you want to say, and what the "facts" tend to show about it.

This is what is meant by "making the case" for and against your hypotheses, and why terms like "argument" are just as relevant here as they are in fields like law and politics. Those fields involve the same kinds of reasoning processes as does science, by connecting facts and conclusions in systematic ways. All are extensions of the same human capacity to analyze, to break things down into parts, and synthesize by putting the parts together, into meaningful, interrelated clusters or wholes. All of us have the natural capabilities and experiences do this. Like other capacities, our ability to critically analyze varied, and even contradictory, evidence is much improved by practice and use in specific areas where we know a lot, so we should practice doing a lot of it, both on paper and in discussions with other people, when we are involved in action-and-inquiry.

After building our basic, internally clear picture, we can then go on to ask such things as, what will my most intelligent critics say, to question my conclusions and facts? What kinds of evidence can I get to assure myself, and others who understand the situation from my point of view, whether my conclusion is correct? What evidence can I get, that would convince the skeptics? Still, we must remember not to get captured by a tendency to react against our imagined critics. That gives them the initiative, and we may end up using their terms and their categories, instead of our own, and if so, we are already one down in the discussion. I recommend that you start where you are strong, with your own, grounded conclusions, and test them out confidently, being willing to revise and shift your ground, to "get it right," before you take the critics too seriously, even in your own imagination. If you are knowledgeable about the program, community or issue you are studying, and if you use your intuitions and observations that are grounded in experience, there are good chances are that you'll have a solid case for the educated guess that you call your "hypothesis." You'll also be flexible and confident enough to change, on the basis of "the evidence," as you go along, so that after a while, you will come to conclusions and evidence that can stand even tough criticism—because you have criticized them, honestly and toughly, yourself.

It is helpful, moreover, to open your work to others' criticisms—hopefully, to friendly, constructive criticisms—and do so, early in the process of any inquiry. We are all subject to "bias," in the sense that we see the world from a partial, special perspective, shaped and limited by our experiences, as well as filled out and enriched by them. We can learn and gain new insights into our own "facts," new ways of posing our questions, and new ways to state our hypotheses and findings, simply by describing them and talking them through with others. You can learn a lot simply by talking to someone about your conclusions and your evidence, and listening to yourself, because you will very likely say things that you hadn't clearly said before to yourself or written down in your outlines or notes. If you're lucky, you will have someone around who is good at "evocative" discussion—drawing you out, helping you say what you want to say, asking questions where it is unclear, reading it back to you as they understand your meaning. That can be almost anyone—family, friends, work colleagues, or professional researchers and teachers—if they understand what you are trying to do, and want to help you do it, instead of pushing you to follow their pet ideas.

Paradigm choice—some of what is at stake

Facts, conclusions, and arguments are not just isolated items, which we happen to connect with each other. They are always enmeshed in, and parts of, larger patterns and ideas. Our values, our basic assumptions about how things are, the ways we like to work, our political convictions, our sense of the social constraints and freedoms we have in our lives—these and many other things are always influencing the hypotheses we come up with, and the "facts" we see and use in our arguments. Many of these we can't do much about; they are just parts of who we are, or our situation at the moment. But some we can choose, and we should think about what our choices mean.

We may, for example, be committed to the conclusion that a program in which we work is doing its job well, though we have yet to do a formal evaluation that will prove it to ourselves and others. We can't choose, at the moment, to ignore or be neutral on that question. But we can choose the whole way we look at what our program's jobs are, and how achievement of its goals is to be defined, and what the most important goals are. We can also look at what we should use as evidence of achievement, how we can argue our case, what counter-arguments and evidence we can discuss, and what "tone" we might best use in approaching the task. This is another example of the importance of Kuhn's use of the term "paradigm" to describe complexes of basic concepts, assumptions, ways of studying a thing, and examples of proved conclusions (Kuhn, 1970). So, our choices of which paradigms, to use make a lot of difference to the direction and content of our action-and-inquiry.

Just as there is no great "Scientific Method" in the sky, that is the correct one, so there is no one way to describe or categorize what we want to study, or the conclusions we want to reach. So, we choose what is at least a crude, beginning approximation, of a paradigm, for each inquiry, whether we do so consciously or not. There is no pre-existing, proven and given, way that we have to think about our program, mission, the desired "outcomes," or current set of significant circumstances. There also is no true version, "out there," somewhere, to be discovered by us, for no other reason that there is never any true and final one. Still, arguably, there are better and worse versions, and ways to go about finding and building better ones. *The criteria or considerations we use to arrive at what's better are debatable, but we can at the very least try to be conscious and clear with ourselves, and also transparent with others, about how we decided what's "better."*

It helps, at least, to have our perspective or "paradigm"—our valued assumptions and considerations consciously in mind, because we, and often others, will live with the consequences of our choices—for better and for worse. Therefore, we do have a lot of freedom to pick our tentative conclusions, and our facts and arguments, to fit the values and purposes we want to serve. It should be added that if we wish our action-and-inquiry to be truly transformative, then we also have the challenge of intermittently re-evaluating our values and purposes, and our overall "paradigm" by seeking out "new" information and by considering fresh and new ways of looking at the data.

If you adopt the transformative approach to action research, you will have already made a commitment to a lot of things that will affect the process and the results. This includes commitments to an openness of your early observations, working descriptively, and diversifying your sampling, and being ready to revise your early conclusions as you go along. You'll keep reaching for conclusions that you hope are true, but still be clear about the evidence against them also. For example, if you're evaluating a school or agency's program, you will be looking for ways of describing and explaining your program's achievements that have the best "fit" with the facts that you observe and that others can observe about the program. In addition, you'll want to keep working for brief, concise, and richly communicative concepts, to make that "fit" as sharp and colorful, and as relevant and apt as possible. This is not a matter of pretty words, and especially not flowery phrases, but of what Albert Einstein has called "naturalness" and "logical simplicity" in the "basic concepts and the relations between them," which he says are important characteristics of a good theory (Schlipp, 1959, p. 23). This is a thing that some mathematicians call "elegance," in the way that concepts are stated and combined, and it is very hard to define clearly. But it's worth reaching for, in formulating, revising, working out your own conclusions and arguments.

Indeed, you may find that the basic way of framing an issue in research is the most powerful single "argument" for or against the evidence being accepted and understood as true *and meaningful*. A basic conception and argument that are simple, internally coherent, and clear may be especially inspiring and persuasive.

Such concepts give us a new way of looking at the setting, community, or program being studied, based on real knowledge of it, and capturing something about its meaning and possibilities that perhaps no one has quite managed to capture in such a compelling way before. And if that kind of newly stated, concise version is richly grounded in the specifics of the setting's or organization's actuality, it may have that "click" effect, which gets an instant response of recognition from people who also know the situation or group or community personally—a sort of "of course, this makes sense; this way of thinking about it, really does 'fit' with the facts." Others will recognize the aptness of this way of explaining and analyzing the topic of action and study, before and underneath their consideration of the formal data and arguments about it. Consequently, the basic vision and message you want to convey will already be more than half conveyed. This is partly because the knowledgeable audience, on reading or hearing such an apt formulation, cranks in a whole complex of their own background "evidence," much of it unconscious, much of it not yet captured in words and perhaps not yet brought out into the arena of discussion. Again, this is not accomplished by fancy words, or PR, or mystification by clever persuasion, but the product of hard work at thinking, and talking, and revising your ideas, in the context of real, personal knowledge about what you are describing and also explaining.

In the same way, your observations, or the comments of participants in a community or group, if they are seen as potential sources of evidence, will often suggest versions of your program and its goals of which you may not have been fully aware. These can then be formulated, discussed, and tested against further evidence. Consider the experience and resulting insight of a nurse in an East Bay community clinic, who realized, during an evaluative discussion of client progress, that by helping one client, a 90-year-old lady walk to the doctor, the nurse not only got the lady to the doctor's office for the first time in a year, but also gave her the first chance in that year to see the flowers and grass and trees that grow along the streets on the way. This, she realized, is "data" about the kind of achievement that her clinic is working for, and it also suggests a new way of describing one clinic goal—the improvement of the quality of life for its community members, going well beyond the usual definitions of "curing illnesses." This analysis of goals, and evidence about their achievement, is now available to that clinic for discussion, in a new way, as parts of their "evaluation efforts."

Barclay Hudson, in his paper "Domains of Evaluation," has suggested some similar considerations in consciously choosing our paradigms for action research (Hudson, 1975). If we want to emphasize specific purposes, to help our communities, and to further certain values, such as more humane public services, we should consciously include those values in our study designs, and pay attention, in data-gathering, to the values inherent in the ways that people treat each other, while pursuing program goals. Some actions, while valuably undertaken for purposes outside themselves, have their own significant meaning, as well—as the way that the nurse walking the lady to the doctor, in the example above, had value beyond its original purpose of getting her there.

Hudson suggests also that we choose paradigms with a clear awareness of whether they focus attention on "strategic variables," things in the situation that people can do something about. This means, partly, defining our concepts, and even what we are studying in the broadest sense, with an eye to what difference it will make for action. It also means, however, not being too guided by what others have taken as the limits of the possible, not confined to the limits of "received theory," in deciding what can be done.

In summary, we should try to be aware of the important elements of our own "paradigm" or primary paradigms. What basic features of our approach to action and research and to our work are most important in shaping the conclusions we come to? The kinds of data we see, and the data we may not notice? The kinds of arguments we make? What are the strong points of our inclinations in these regards? What constraints are we possibly assuming that we must accept, that we might get free of, if we think about all this some more?

Figuring out what "evidence" to have confidence in

So far, I have emphasized the importance of the guiding paradigm you choose, the conclusions you set out to verify or test, and the building of a meaningful picture out of your data and your conclusions. I said that the way a concept fits the available data is one test of its worth and usefulness, but that other things, like its "elegance" and "logical simplicity," and the purposes that it serves in social action, are also important in assessing it. Similarly, in testing the value of any piece of "evidence," we may look at the degree to which it makes sense as a part of the meaningful picture we are building, composed of conclusions and evidence for and against them. That means it may be more valuable if it fits in, and helps, fill out the picture more richly and understandably. However, *evidence also may be useful if it is dissonant, if it seems relevant, but doesn't somehow "go" with the other parts of the picture.* That piece of evidence may be the key to something deeply wrong with our picture, or only to a minor revision that will give us an "ah-ha" experience more tellingly, once we understand what the dissonance is about.

Besides the "fit" of "pieces" of evidence with conclusions, we can pose other tests to our observations and the comments of others. Some people, trained in the tradition of "hard" science as the only science there is, despair of there being any meaningful social or historical research that is worthy of the name. In such matters, they believe, everything is "simply a matter of opinion," and one opinion is just about as good as another. That is one reason why so many social scientists in trying to get beyond "opinions" then resort to numbers, based on counts of "behavioral" indicators, supposedly bypassing variations in human interpretation. But consider the following scenario.

Suppose you are studying something like the state of working relationships in a community organization, and you begin to get indications that there is a standing tension between staff and higher administration, which is getting in the way of the agency's doing its job well. How would it affect your acceptance of this "piece of data":

—if one of the people working in the agency told you it was so?

—if several different people who work there told you the same thing?

—if several people told you the same thing, and they have different jobs or positions in the agency, which carry different experiences of its operations?

—if several people told you, and they have tended to differ on other things, such as their political convictions, age, backgrounds, and the like?

—if several people told you the same thing, and they have different structural positions in the organization, such as "staff" and "higher administration" and "board"?

—if several people told you, and they have different interests in the truth of the statement, such as the person in charge of public relations, the custodian, and the leading spokesperson for "staff" points of view?

—if the people who tell you have some special reason to know—such as special access to meetings where the conflicts have been talked about, or expertise in understanding work-relationships, or a reputation among their co-workers for being informed, honest observers?

—if the people telling you appear to have some special motives in telling you—such as making themselves look good, or maintaining an "everything is OK" picture of the organization, or pushing their own, special view of what the organization ought to be doing, or how it does it?

What if people disagree, and some of your informants seem to you to have more thoughtful, subtle ways of looking at things in general—not all right/wrong, black/white, simple and definite, but more processual, textured, and careful about small things that may be important? What if that appearance to you is backed up by what people in the agency tell you about each other? What if, not only are you told this datum by people working in the agency, but you personally observe people there acting in ways consistent with what they have told you? What if these observations and the comments of others are not just a one-time thing, but a recurrent feature of the agency, as you go back to visit it several times? What if other things about the place change over time, but this one seems to stay relatively constant?

In other words: How would each of these possibilities affect your confidence in the notion that the agency had a bad staff/management split, and conflict problem? Would several of them, together, prove it? Would they make you think it's probably true? What would be enough for you to put it in your research, as a datum or one of your conclusions? What else would affect your accepting this conclusion? How would you test to see if that conclusion is right?

These are some of the kinds of issues that you will encounter, continually, in doing action research on real community programs in real agencies. If you pay attention to them, and to others that you develop for yourself as you go along, you are not very likely to come out saying that "one opinion is as good as another," or that you have 100% certainty about any one of your conclusions, or pieces of evidence. Instead, you will find that some data and conclusions are a lot better than others, that you can feel quite confident, until proven wrong, about some of your conclusions, and that you are doing very deliberately a kind of research that flows naturally out of the ways you understand the world as you walk through it, every day.

You will likely find, not that all opinions are equally valid, but that people tell you different, and conflicting, things, about some aspects of their organization's or community's life. Some of us call this the "Rashomon effect," after the famous Japanese film, in which several different people tell persuasive, but sharply conflicting, stories about a murder in the forest. When you hit this situation where people have very different interpretations of the "facts," this is where some of these methods action-and-inquiry can be very helpful, even if you are never certain about "the conclusion."

As one strategy, we can sometimes zero in on what facts and conclusions to have confidence in by doing what is called "cross-validation," or "triangulation." This means that we can improve the validity of our findings by getting not only different people's comments, but also different kinds of evidence on the same issue. For example, if we not only get comments from people saying that there is staff conflict, but we also observe it—and perhaps also find references to it in official memos, or observe little subtle things about the ways people act and how the place feels tense to us, or learn that past projects have been abandoned for lack of cooperation. Such different sources and qualities of evidence will likely make us more confident that we are right. Of course, we may rarely have anything so clear as to have all of these indicators pointing the same way, but we can work with the data we have, and if a couple of types of data seem to confirm one another, then this is often quite enough for the purposes at hand.

Validity and reliability: Two different emphases in weighing the evidence

Among professional researchers, and many other people as well, the problem of differences in research results is a major concern. Different people may report different observations about the same situation, or what seem to be similar situations. They may even present different interpretations of the same body of established "facts." What do these differences mean? What kinds of research approaches can be taken to address them?

Two different emphases have grown up in social research, to dealing with this recurring problem. As discussed earlier, one approach, emphasizing what is called "reliability" of results, lays a heavy reliance on standardizing the procedures used in gathering and analyzing data, to assure that any two researchers, using those procedures, will get very similar results when studying the same or similar situations. For example, IQ tests, and even more recently developed and sophisticated psychological tests, have been developed this way, and they are said to be very "reliable," because the same person will get very similar scores, no matter how often they take the same test, or similar tests. The procedures used to build reliability here involve the use of standardized, quantifiable lists of questions or items, and developing agreed-on definitions for what specific, numerical scores (numbers of "right" answers) on these questions mean. This approach to the issue of different facts and interpretations seems to "solve" the "problem" by eliminating differences before they can happen. The big source of uniformity in this method is in the procedures used to study the situation.

These procedures structure and define the data and their interpretations down to lists of simple items, which are then added up, to give clear, well-defined and very precise results. From each person's definite score on the IQ tests, the researchers then infer a similarly definite "level" of "intelligence."

By contrast, those who emphasize what is called "validity," approach the differences in facts and interpretations, not by immediately considering these seeming contradictions or inconsistencies as a "problem" to be "solved." Instead, those inquiring see these differences in the data, as points of departure for trying to understand better what is being studied, that is, for trying to get at the reality behind the different formulations. Instead of starting out with highly standardized procedures for studying "intelligence," for example, this approach tends to have us ask such things as, "what is 'intelligence,' anyway? What different observations have people made, about their own and others' intelligence?" How can we account for different observations about the intelligence of a single person? How do different people demonstrate "intelligence"? What can our different observations tell us about the thing we call "intelligence?"

For those of us who emphasize "validity," our concern is for getting at the reality below the surface of whatever we are studying, realizing that our first versions of what we are studying may not even be stated properly. We may start by asking: What is intelligence? But we may later decide that this is not the issue, but some other question that we could not think of at first. We might, decide, for example, that different types of "competence" are more relevant to our interests, or more useful in getting at what we want to know about, than the subject of "intelligence," in general.

These two emphases might be illustrated by considering a well-known story—the one about the blind men and the elephant. As the story goes, a group of blind men approach an elephant. One feels the elephant's trunk and declares the animal must be a snake. Another feels its ear, and says that the animal is flat and thin, like a very sturdy leaf. Another feels a leg and says the animal must certainly look like a tree. A fourth feels the tail, and says the animal seems to be very much like a rope. The message of the story is that all of us are in the predicament of not immediately being able to observe and "validly" make conclusions about any reality we are studying. Different people make different observations and formulate different interpretations of the same thing. The famous story ends there, but let's take it a step further.

The researcher who emphasizes reliability of data would tend to come to the blind men's rescue by giving them a standardized procedure for making their observations. He might get them all to line up at one place, let's say the elephant's trunk. One after another, each blind man would step forward and feel the trunk. This procedure would successfully eliminate all disagreement. The blind men would unanimously conclude that the elephant is really a snake, or at least seems to be very much like a thick snake. This is reliability, but at the expense of validity. We have created a method to get consistency among observations and interpretations, at the expense of an accurate understanding of reality, which is invariably quite complex.

The researcher who emphasizes validity might instead urge the blind men to wander about the elephant's body. They might say, "don't feel this animal at any one place, roam all over him." Find out what the parts, and the boundaries, of him are. Talk to each other, compare observations, and discuss your differences. If one of you feels he has a snake here, call to the one who feels a tree and say, "Tree stump, huh? Well, what does this long, round, wriggling thing feel like to you?" Then the two of you can try to find your way back to part that felt like a tree trunk that one person felt, and while you are on the way, see what else you feel.

This research method is much closer to the approach we are urging. This is "exploration" or a conscious effort to "broaden our experiences" of what we are studying. We are trying to get a diverse sample, to observe a *variety* of parts and connections that make up the "elephant." This is inquiry with an emphasis on validity, trying to find out what a *complicated* reality is all about. It is a process, not a single, standard set of procedures that can be set out with no ambiguity. It involves ingenuity, and common sense, and wandering all about, and comparing notes with others, and critiquing and building on our first ideas as we go. It's not aimless wandering, but alert and very purposive wandering, figuring out how to get more and better information, and trying not to miss too much as we go. It is *a messier process* than the one chosen by those experts whose main emphasis is reliability, but it also helps us in avoiding the error of unanimous agreement about a very wrong and useless (or sometimes destructive) conclusion. In addition, once we begin to get a coherent, valid picture of our "elephant," our reliability will increase; that is, we will eventually begin to agree with one another about the shape and appearance of what we are observing and noticing. But, this time, our agreed-on picture will be a more accurate reflection of reality.

The dialectic of thought and action

(Revised and updated from an earlier paper with Dr. Terry Lunsford.)

Both thought and action have important roles in action research. Many versions of action research see "action" to be the consequence of "research." First, one does research, and then, based on the information and ideas obtained during the research, one formulates some recommendations and directions for action which are then implemented. This view does not fully acknowledge the dynamic interplay and intermixing of action and research.

The transformative approach to action research emphasizes the dialectic of thought and action. By dialectic, I mean a kind of relationship between thought and action, which calls attention to the potential of each to transform the other. Through action we can generate new ideas, modify and refine "old" ideas and theories, and generally improve our thinking. Through reflection on our action, we can gain new insights into the significance of our action—of the values served, the various ("positive" and "negative") outcomes, as well as possibilities and alternatives for future action. Action can serve as a vehicle for transforming and improving our thinking and our ideas, while critical and inquisitive thinking can lead to a transformation of our daily practices and planned actions, helping us to learn from experience and pointing the way for our subsequent actions.

Sometimes, the flow of our everyday activities is such that we do not take a lot of time for thinking and reflection. We will, of course, have "thoughts" about our actions, but we may not do much in the way of probing and systematic reflection into their meaning and significance. Saul Alinsky, the famous community organizer, once noted that he valued those periods of time he had spent in jail, because it was then when he was able to take the time to "stand back" from the incessant rush of community organizing activity and reflect on his strategies. In jail, he was able to evaluate strategies, and conceptualize and write about theories of community organizing based on his previous activities.

One aim of this book is to help you to develop methods and strategies for critically reflecting on your actions without having to go into self-imposed exile, or to wait for those periods when you are out of commission, whether it be in the hospital, in jail, exhausted at home from burnout, or sheltering at home during a pandemic. It's good for all of us to think about how we can build continual opportunities for thought and reflection into the flow of our everyday activities.

It is equally important to develop strategies to provide opportunities to experiment with new courses of action. Action is an important part of inquiry. The conventional academician must wait for action to "happen" and then build theory from the actions of others. By contrast, those of us involved in change and improvement efforts, in *action research* have interests and opportunities to create action, which we can then use to test out our ideas, refine our thinking and practices, and explore unknown areas of concern. Through action we can generate situations which may not previously have existed, or which previously were quite removed from our own experiences, as a way of exploring or testing out our ideas. If we are interested in preventive health care and community participation in setting agency practices and policies aimed at such health care, we might choose to set up a clinic, or a new program that would explore these ideas. Instead of looking around to see if some clinic is already doing this, and then being frustrated by the absence of information because such clinics are few and far between, we might decide to test these ideas out for ourselves by setting up such a clinic or program.

When I was teaching at the University of Cincinnati in the College of Community Services, I noted that most students were frustrated and distracted from significant learning because would spend all their time running from one activity to another, among their many classes and field placement. Consequently, they ended up going through the motions in each activity. They didn't have time to think deeply about the significance of these activities, and this limited their learning. Even their field placements became just another activity, another course to "complete" satisfactorily. The structure and scheduling of all these activities didn't allow students to explore their interests in depth, nor to create and experiment with new activities and to reflect on their experiences.

I proposed to the faculty that we loosen this structure, but still with guidance, to give students the space to do this kind of exploration, experimentation, and critical reflection. Most faculty took the position that there was no evidence to indicate that my proposal would work, so I pointed out that in the absence of trying it out we would have no way of knowing whether or not it would work, but that there was a lot of evidence to indicate that the existing arrangement was far from ideal. Eventually, with my colleague, Harry Butler, we were able to successfully lobby for the creation of an experimental program to test out these ideas—an experiment which was an example of taking action both to test out an idea and to generate new ideas, as well as a worthwhile action in and of itself.

That experimental program did point out the general validity of the methods used, although, given the politics of the University, the College did not adopt that strategy for all students. Nor did all the faculty agree about the value of the experiment, and each had their different interpretations of the "data" or the "experience" about the experiment—a point relevant to the previous discussion on "making sense out of our experiences" and "judging the evidence." More significantly, however, from the views of those participating, the experimental program had a profound impact on those faculty, students, and community service workers who were highly involved with it. For many of us, including Harry Butler and myself, the actions and experiences that were part of that experiment transformed our thinking and our future actions. We refined our understanding of how learning takes place, improved our own methods of teaching and learning, and came to some new insights about teaching, learning, action research, and community work.

Such examples point out that action can be an important way to test out theory, and also to refine, or even develop, theory and future practice/action. In discussing "praxis," which is a concept for the dialectic of thought and action, Barclay Hudson points out in his article "Domains of Evaluation" that:

> The question of "what ought to be done" is very much a reflection of what you think *can* be done. And what can be done is not a belief that springs from what now seems possible but from a higher-level question:
>
> *"Can you make the world possible to do this?"* When social program evaluation asks that kind of question, it enters the fifth domain of praxis that we are talking about. (Hudson, 1975)

The whole question of "what is possible?" is not an easy one—it is not merely a "logical" extension of past experience or available data, nor merely a matter of one's hopes and commitments, but part of a more intricate logic. That logic involves the dialectic of thought and action, and values, purposes, and commitments are of course part of the thought and the action, as well.

8

COMMUNICATING AND COLLABORATING

Although people often think of communicating one's findings and taking action to be the last step in doing action research, they sometimes are also the beginning of further action-inquiry. Some people may repeat the various steps in the research process—asking questions, gathering data, analyzing data, communicating findings (thus far), and taking action—continually and for an extended period of time. This is especially the case when we find ourselves trying to address some similar problems and pursue some similar purposes and concerns for a very long period of time. In the previous section on "The dialectic of thought and action" I discussed how thought can, often does, contribute to action, and likewise, action can lead to deeper, more insightful thoughts.

This chapter is a further discussion of the important role of collaboration in transformative action-and-inquiry. As was previously discussed, collaboration is extremely important in science and all research—natural sciences, academic social sciences, and action research. Sharing ideas with one another and soliciting their participation and contributions almost always greatly improve the quality of our inquiry. Further, we must communicate to, and share with, others the details of the process that led to our findings. By being transparent about how we have arrived at our findings, others can make well-informed decisions about how seriously to take those findings, and potentially they can contribute to our next steps to test out, revise, and further develop our findings and ideas. Finally, collaboration is also important and valuable when taking action. *This chapter is about three related considerations—how to best communicate what we know to others, how and why we should collaborate with others to improve our research and our action, and how to provide transparency about how we have arrived at our findings.*

The role of collaboration in action research and inquiry

Collaboration should be, and often is, an integral part of every stage of the research process and contributes to creative and effective research. It is not surprising that many Noble Prizes are awarded to more than one person, to colleagues or a team. The following research on American scientists found that Noble laureates were much more likely to collaborate (Zuckerman, 1967) https://www.jstor.org/stable/2091086?seq=1#page_scan_tab_contents/ Interestingly, however, the article also found that they collaborated less after receiving the award perhaps because "The prize generates strain in collaborative associations so that most of these terminate soon after the award." It would seem that collaboration may be an extremely valuable quality to nurture, despite, and in the face of, the unfortunate, competitive pressures that exist in many societies.

Collaborating with others is also an important step to increase transparency about our research methods and helps us and others to be more aware and conscious of our role in making judgments during the research process. At its best, inquiry is not something done by a single person in isolation, but a continuing process that involves cooperation and collaboration between two or more people. In terms of social change, community improvement and institutional reform, collaboration not only enhances the quality of the knowledge-building and insights that ensue but also is often essential to putting knowledge into action. Knowledge without active citizen participation is, at best limited, unfulfilled potential, and at worst, worthless. In the transformative approach to action-and-inquiry, community knowledge-building (see Chapter 12) is exceedingly important, for example, in developing "community action think tanks," where groups of people from all walks of life might come together to wrestle with challenging problems, hoping for new insights for feasible, change-producing actions.

Even in the realm of the so-called "hard sciences," "ordinary people" have the capability of making important contributions. For example, when *Discover Magazine* reported on the 2010s top 100 science stories, one story was "Scientists tap wisdom of crowds" (Cavalier, 2011, p. 74):

> When University of Washington biochemist David Baker needed help predicting the structure of proteins, he did not turn to his colleagues. Rather, he decided to let the whole world participate. Increasingly, scientists are relying on such "crowdsourcing"—calling on ordinary citizens to volunteer their help in addressing complicated problems. In Baker's case, he helped develop Foldit, a computer game that challenges players to wiggle and shake protein chains into stable structures. In August a paper in Nature revealed that Foldit players, most of whom had little or no biochemical education, surpassed or matched the performance of a sophisticated protein-folding algorithm on 8 of 10 puzzles. "People are better at analyzing the whole situation," Baker says. "Computers just approach problems randomly." Volunteers for the Galaxy Zoo project have classified a million images from the Sloan Digital Sky Survey, leading to about 20 scientific publications and one genuine enigma: a peculiar green intergalactic blob. Other crowdsourced projects include labeling aerial photos of Mongolia in a quest to find Genghis Khan's tomb and improving climate models by pouring over World War I ship logs for weather information. Government agencies are getting in on

the action too, listing projects on a new Web site, Challenge.gov, and offering prizes. In July a retired engineer from New Hampshire won $30,000 from NASA for a model that forecast solar activity with 75 percent accuracy. "There's a huge appetite from people who aren't scientists to actually involved in science," says Galaxy Zoo principal investigator Chris Lintott.

Soliciting broader participation in inquiry and research isn't only about increasing the "quantity" of labor in hopes that one or two people will have a conceptual breakthrough or stumble onto a "hidden" piece of data. The old saying "two heads are better than one," is quite true, and collaboration provides many different opportunities for improving the breadth and depth of inquiry. In the realm of social change and community improvement, collaboration improves the quality of inquiry and contributes to the citizen participation essential in a democratic society. The importance, and interconnectedness of these principles can be found in the work of two well-known scholar-activists discussed in Chapter 3—John Dewey (Dewey, 1968) and Paulo Freire (Freire, 1972).

As another example, many of us may have had the personal experience of pairing off with a friend, and then asking one another evocative questions. In thinking about and trying to articulate answers or comments, we often come up with new insights and new ways of saying out loud whatever it is that we're trying to understand better and then write about. This is a valuable example of how two students can help each other to write papers or theses and overcome difficulties in getting the right words down on a piece of paper. For instance, one student can come up with the key questions that they wish to address, and then have their friend "quiz them"—and the friend can probe, and ask for expansion, clarification, and illuminating examples.

Inquiry and others, learning from and with others—"collaboration"

(Revised and updated from an earlier paper with Dr. Terry Lunsford.)

Inquiry and others

Thus far, I have mostly focused on our various individual ways of engaging in inquiry. How do we experience and observe our community work? How do we analyze and make sense out of our experiences? How do we judge and evaluate evidence pertaining to our community work and activities? I have noted that our approaches to the collection, interpretation, evaluation, and uses of data will vary according to our own interests and to our needs, purposes and prior experiences. Inevitably, there will also be individual differences in our efforts to inquire into particular circumstances and situations. Still, I've also emphasized some general principles and considerations, which can be kept in mind as we go about the task of making our action research valid and useful.

Now, I wish to emphasize that *while each person's inquiry should be shaped in part by their individual needs and purposes, research in general and action research in particular should be seen as a social process. Further, at its best, research involves collaboration.* It involves people comparing notes, testing out their ideas with one another, critiquing and listening to each other's observations, and carefully considering each other's interpretations and approaches to weighing the evidence. Collaboration involves several types of cooperative effort, including 1) listening to one another to try to learn from the other's ideas, experiences, observations, and methods of inquiry; 2) giving the other person constructive criticism to point out things they may be overlooking or overemphasizing; 3) trying to create ideas and actions which are much more significant, useful, and worthwhile than what could be created by any one person by themselves.

Remember the story in Chapter 7 about the blind men and the elephant. In order to increase the likelihood of having a "valid" finding, the blind men needed to compare notes, to talk with each other, to discuss what they were finding out with each other, and to give each other suggestions about new directions for exploring and "making sense of the experiences" the elephant.

Collaboration acknowledges that we live in the world together, and that our world is a social world in many important respects. Therefore, our research and action must also be seen as part of a social process.

Learning from others

When we are embarking on a new project, it is often useful for us to stop and ask ourselves, what can we learn from others? What kinds of things might we find out from others, who, by virtue of their special experiences or insights, might be able to help illuminate the action and/or research we are contemplating? For example, we can often learn a lot from the successes and failures of others. Are there some projects similar to ours? What problems did they encounter? Are there one or two projects that seemed to have some special noteworthy successes where others failed? We will not necessarily want to copy the methods employed by those who were successful, nor will we necessarily decide to avoid all the practices pursued by those who "failed" or had difficulties. Nevertheless, consideration of related efforts made by others can be informative and point the way to some issues and concerns of which we will want to be very much aware as we proceed.

The traditional version of this concern for learning from others sometimes takes the form of a "review of the literature." Often, researchers will begin by doing an exhaustive search for articles and books on the topic to be studied. Unfortunately, some of these efforts are primarily for appearances—to prove to professional colleagues that one is aware of the relevant research and prepared to defend their findings against the backdrop of that other research. This can take on the quality of one-ups-man-ship. But approached in a different way, an examination of books and articles related to one's area of concern can be used as one good way of learning from others. Critique the articles, not to make a point, or put down the other person—but critique the articles as a way of sharpening one's own perspective. How are my purposes and concerns different from others who have done inquiry into a similar area? How are they similar? Have others looked at different "facts" than I am inclined to? If so, why? Am I missing something important, and/or are they giving undue consideration to some things while neglecting other important concerns? Through such questioning, it is possible to become more aware of one's own perspectives—biases, if you wish—and then to evaluate critically the strengths and weaknesses of those guiding perspectives.

Further, it is not always necessary to do a review of the literature *before* "beginning" to do research. Sometimes this may be very appropriate and helpful, and at other times, it may be best to start by immersing oneself in the project, by going "where the action is" and then later comparing one's observations and experiences with what others have to say in their writings.

Of course, books and papers are not the only source of learning from others. One may choose to do formal or informal interviews with others who have been involved in related projects, as was touched on in Chapter 6. One may collect oral histories from people who have experienced a particular situation or set of social conditions for an extended period of time. If, for example, we are going to study preventive health care, we might wish not only to review professional health journals, but also perhaps to take oral histories of people who have lived long and healthy lives. What have their lives been like? What have been their health practices, the conditions in their environment and social surroundings, and so forth? We may wish to interview people who themselves have been involved in successful, and not so successful, programs aimed at preventive health care. From such combinations of reading and talking with others, we may be able to develop a number of interesting case studies—about individual people, about groups of people, about special programs. These case studies may point out issues to consider as we continue to pursue our own action research efforts.

Very often, it is quite informative to consider the experiences of people in different cultures, or in strikingly different social circumstances. By trying to learn from those in markedly different contexts, we may get important insights from the similarities and differences among those experiences. Continuing with the previous example, if we consider preventive health efforts in different countries, or issues of preventive health among wealthy vs. impoverished classes of people in our own society, we may learn a lot about the nature of preventive health.

Collaboration is also important to action in community work. It is a way of getting people involved, of helping people to explore their concerns and interests together. It is a way of making inquiry happen—of questioning, of doing critical thinking about observations, and of discussing different judgments in light of data and values. All of this can be part of one's everyday work and life. Collaboration is the principal vehicle through which participation gets built into research within an organization or community group. This participation will improve the quality of the inquiry, whether it is day-to-day discussion of how to improve agency practices, a major year-end program evaluation, a needs assessment, a staff-board planning retreat, or a way to strengthen the group's effectiveness in reaching out to others in the community. Furthermore, as an end in itself, collaborative inquiry can facilitate participation within an organization, and also serve to involve people outside the organization (e.g., clients, students, community constituents or prospective board members) in the activities of the organization.

As an exercise, you might want to try to apply informally some of these ideas about collaboration to see what you can learn by this cooperative approach to inquiry. For example, test out some important observations or ideas with someone whom you think may have some different, but still potentially valuable, ways of looking at these ideas. Question and critique some of their ideas or observations. Can the two (or several) of you come up with some observations, ideas, or issues worth further inquiry that go beyond what any of you could have come up with by yourselves?

A special kind of collaboration that is often useful in doing action research is collaboration between people with different roles. For example, staff, clients, and board members often have different perspectives on activities in their organization, in part because of their different roles. Staff with different positions—e.g., different levels and types of authority and responsibility—are also likely to have different experiences within the agency and different ways of interpreting and evaluating agency activities.

Collaboration between people with different roles can be especially illuminating because these people are likely to suggest to one another different ways of looking at things. Also, they may have access to different kinds of information. Secretaries often have access to all kinds of informal gossip, and hear about frustrations and concerns, that sometimes fall outside the knowledge and experience of an agency director. By contrast, agency directors sometimes know more details about the politics involved with funding agencies. This is not to say that the secretary should have the final say about interpreting the meaning and significance of gossip nor should the director have the final word on interpreting the implications of the politics with external agencies. But each one can learn a lot from the other. Each can contribute information, and the other one can bring a fresh perspective and important questions to interpreting and evaluating that which is "news" to them. Potentially they can get a lot of insights by collaborating with each other.

Board members can be especially helpful if they are used as "friendly critics," as people who know something about the agency and are sympathetic to its purposes, but who are not as wrapped up in day-to-day activities as staff are. For this reason, they can often ask hard questions and raise important issues, whereas sometimes staff who are heavily involved with everyday work may lose sight of some issues and questions that need to be considered. This is especially true if board members are given opportunities to stay in touch with what's going on, if they are informed, and if they can observe agency activities and have opportunities to confer with staff.

All of this is to say that *collaboration between different people—especially between people with different roles, experiences, and values, assuming perhaps a general level of goodwill and some shared sense of purpose—can be very helpful to action research.* Collaboration is a way of testing out our observations, and our analyses and evaluations of data. It is one important safeguard against our coming up with observations and judgments, which are merely subjective, or narrowly biased.

Learning with others

Collaboration involving learning with others is of course a more intense kind of involvement and a more fully cooperative effort than the learning from others described above. This kind of collaboration is especially suited to co-workers. We can use ongoing, informal dialogue and conversation with our co-workers as an integral part of action research. It is possible to compare observations with each other, to test out hypotheses, to discuss each other's evaluations of actions taken, and more.

Part of the success of ongoing informal collaboration depends on the nature of the day-to-day working and interpersonal relationships. If there is a spirit of trust and cooperation, a genuinely shared desire to learn from each other, and therefore to learn with each other, then much can be accomplished informally. Still, it is necessary to exert the effort and take the time to discuss issues of mutual interest on a regular basis, and to have the self-discipline to question one another, to raise issues and challenge one another in a supportive atmosphere.

It's much like the self-discipline of cross-country running—two teammates run together and practice together not so that one can outdistance the other, but so that each will push and encourage the other to go faster and to exert more effort, and perhaps to get into a nice "rhythm." A significant difference, of course, is that action research involves striving for qualitatively deeper insights, not just a quantitative increase in effort or "output." Beyond this, it should be added that people often enjoy the experience of running with a friend, and indeed, collaboration in many areas can be quite stimulating and enjoyable.

There are also formalized ways of pursuing such collaboration within one's community organization. There can be regularly scheduled meetings for staff to share ideas. Some meetings may be billed as brainstorming sessions, while others may be focused group discussions on specific issues. Some meetings may be devoted to sharing observations related to a certain area of concern, while other sessions may be all-day retreats to make decisions about issues, which have been discussed on a regular basis for quite some time. Other meetings may be structured as "group interviews" with one staff member interviewing others as a way of eliciting ideas and information from them on some topic(s) of concern.

Communicating what we know to others

(Revised and updated from an earlier paper with Dr. Terry Lunsford.)
Just as working through an inquiry is best made a process of collaboration with others, communicating what we know from our research is a shared process, a social interaction, with our audiences. Getting into that process early in our inquiry

will have made it a lot easier for us to communicate what it's all about when we are through. So, we should talk about what we are learning from our action research, frequently, with friends and colleagues, as we are doing the action research. For now, however, I want us to concentrate on the task of writing up what we want to say about the research-action. Unfortunately, for many sharp, articulate people, writing, especially about something important, often feels like a special problem. It needn't be. In my own experience, high school courses and college courses in writing were of little help, and mostly were demoralizing for me. I lost confidence that I could ever write well, and only in graduate school did I have the good fortune of benefiting from the supportive and informal instruction of several people. So, even though I know I must continue to work on improving my writing, I no longer feel inhibited and anxious about it. I'll talk more about this later in this chapter.

One important thing, as stated above, is to start writing early. Before we start "gathering data," when we are figuring out what we want to do, we should write versions of it down, however briefly, and let others look at what we've written. It will help us to formulate our thoughts more systematically and give others a clear and definite enough of an idea of what we are doing so that they can give us good feedback and suggestions. Most of all, *we'll probably find that, as we write things down, new ideas come to us, and we will realize that we are thinking things that we hadn't quite said to ourselves until we started to write. Sometimes, it is helpful to record ourselves speaking and then listen to what we said and take notes then.*

Write to ourselves, first. Make sense to ourselves, before we worry about other people. Especially if, writing feels awkward or scary, we should try writing a lot—but only for our own eyes, so we can get our writing muscles loosened up, without the fearfulness of knowing that others will see and judge what we've written. Some of the best writers in history have been people who wrote and re-wrote, over and over, before they got it "right." We needn't be ashamed of many messy notes and scratched-over drafts, if that's how we find that we like or need to work. The point is, we should do whatever helps us to get our thoughts down coherently, or even just very roughly at first.

We should try to be tolerant of doing many, tentative versions of what we are writing, but make each of them as little work as possible. With practice, we can find what feels comfortable, and natural, to our own style of thinking and working. We can put down notes on ideas, for example, whenever we think of them. By noting down the nub of an idea, we can then later come back and expand it into something more elaborate. Or we can sometimes sit down, right then, and write a paragraph or so, to get the fullness of the idea into words while it is just aborning in our mind, so to speak, of its own accord. That's often when the flow comes most easily, and the fullness of the idea will almost "tell itself."

As we get well along in our research, we should work over our field notes, every now and then, pulling out of them whatever seem like the most interesting ideas, the best pieces of evidence, the most unexpected findings, the strongest conclusions. These are starts on making sense out of the data, in terms we can communicate to others, and the earlier and more often we do it, usually the better.

We needn't get trapped into feeling that we must start with the first page and write straight through to the last—or not start at all. We can start at many places: the one biggest conclusion we are reaching for, the heart of our analysis of the data; the framework setting part of the introduction; or whatever flows best at the time. If we start early, and keep at it off and on, we'll have time to draft many parts of it, in chunks. We can pull these chunks together and give them the needed connective tissue, later on, when the shape of the whole has begun to emerge clearly in our mind. Writing parts of it out for ourselves will help that shape to emerge in a way that sometimes nothing else will.

Also, we can search for the "flow"—what gets us writing and making sense—and use whatever crude and partial forms feel most do-able at the time: outlines, paragraphs, rough notes to capture an insight. But we should try to be working, all the time, in the direction of clarity and coherence in making our points, first to ourselves, then to others. It may be useful, after we get started, to keep in mind the idea of some "friendly critics" whom we know, in such a way that we try to write to help them understand what we want to say, and see the conclusions as justified.

As I have repeatedly suggested, start with something that we want to say. *Find what feels right to us, as worth saying, as the version that fits what we know about the thing we have been studying, the story that we think needs telling.* Then, any modifications we make will be from that solid base—and we won't be captured by the demands of powerful audiences whom we may feel we have to reach. Indeed, however, there are some delicate balances to be searched for, in this imagined discourse with our audiences.

Language is part of it. We should focus on writing for ourselves in whatever words and phrases grab out insights and capture them for our later use. Also, when we communicate them to others, we should consciously put them in terms our identified audiences can understand. We should use words they know the meanings of, in the first place—not fancy jargon or "in" phrases that our particular audience of outsiders may not understand. If we want employers or foundation people or government officials or academics to appreciate our research, we may have to avoid "street talk," or slang expressions that will turn them off and make us sound "unprofessional." Even little slips of grammar or punctuation or spelling can sometimes be taken by such readers as indicators of our incompetence, so it's simple sense to get someone who's good at those things to look over our work before the final draft, to clear up the small errors that we may have missed.

Yet, one of the worst effects of that kind of concern with legitimating our writing is that we may try to talk "academese," and use research terms, like "variables" and "standard deviations," or bureaucratic language (like "utilize" instead of "use") and "implement" and "program planning capabilities," when these specialized terms are really unnecessary, and much too abstract to say what really is intended. Terms like that not only mess up the clarity of our writing, but they also get in the way of clear thinking, because they are someone else's language, into which we are trying to fit our concerns because we think we have to. They are much less clear, and have much less meaning, than the natural, direct, concrete, colorful ways of thinking and talking that engaged, involved people use when dealing with, and communicating about, a subject in which they are interested.

In communicating about action research project results, it can be just as important to put our ideas in terms that non-professionals can understand—our own community board, co-workers, people who don't care so much about official-ese or current buzz-words, but who just want to know what we've discovered and concluded that is worthwhile. Speaking and writing to such audiences often is the best guide to clear and coherent writing. Within that general framework, our own personal variations and writing style can lend a lot of humanness and enjoyability to the reader's task of understanding us. We can check it out with our friendly critics, but *we shouldn't be afraid to say things in ways that are our own, and which capture the feel of what we want people to know.*

Being aware of our audience goes beyond words to tone, content, and implications of what we are saying. We may, in some cases, want our readers to know that we disagree strongly with them—for example, that we are formally protesting the evaluation standards being used to judge our agency's performance. Then, we will want to say so, as respectfully as we feel is honest, but in clear and unmistakable terms that's intentional, and purposive. But we should take care not to slap our audience in the face disrespectfully or unintentionally—by referring to administrators as "bureaucrats," for example, or by assuming that our audience shares our values or political convictions that we have no reason to believe they share, or by lecturing them about the right way to act according to our principles. Also, we should avoid insulting our readers' intelligence, by not over-explaining simple things, and by not "talking down" to them from the height of our moral purity, or our new-found research knowledge. The whole tone of our writing—its implicit assumptions about who is talking, and to whom—needs to be as honest and natural as it can be, faithful to the real situation as we know it, without being unaware of what our actual, intended audiences are going to be like.

If one of your main audiences is likely to be hostile, or merely impersonally skeptical, as is often the case with funding sources and government agencies, you may think that this is the clear case for talking in terms that they can hear, or else their preconceptions will prevent their giving you a fair hearing. For example, sometimes it is very realistic to talk "research talk," in presenting your data and conclusions to a group that you think will have simplistic, traditional views about what "good" research is—very structured, very quantitative, very technical, very jargonized. Sometimes it would be naive and unrealistic to think that you can address such an audience, as you would talk to others who already appreciate and understand this transformative, and often qualitative, approach to action research. On the other hand, you can easily get trapped into trying to talk "their way," and not quite make it, and in the process, lose your faithfulness to the real terms and the real point of your own research efforts. In other words, *the delicate balance does involve a search for some midpoint between naiveté and defensiveness. But I'd urge that you err mostly on the side of risking some naiveté, to be sure that you don't distort your own work and the real message of your research.* In any case, pandering to the terms of the audience's preconceptions, when you don't really respect or like what they stand for, can sap your self-respect, and feed a lack of confidence that you really have something to say, and have used methods for saying it that have worth and solidity in them. This is one of the latent effects of that kind of specialized jargon in many fields—to put you on the defensive because you fear you don't know the "code." This then gives "the insiders" a leg up in any discussion, without regard to the content of their ideas. Instead of becoming a victim of that, it's better to reach for the underlying virtues of good research and good communication as we know them. This means *communicating clear ideas, grounded in direct contact with the things studied, tested against tough objections and alternatives, and explained in simple, strong reasoning.* Those will help you put your *"best foot forward,"* more often than not, without your having to know the right jargon-words for the particular audience in question.

Starting from that position, you can aim to do more than "report" your research to a narrow colleague group and can strive to improve both your research and your communication. You may have to learn to educate your audiences about the importance, the background, and the frame of reference, for understanding what your research is all about. This may mean setting the stage in an introduction, which tells why you did this particular piece of research, why it's important beyond itself, what difference it makes to your community, to your organization, or to broader social-change efforts. Often, audiences outside the setting where you work will know little about that setting, and your way of analyzing it can teach them as much as your data or your conclusions. Also, writing explicitly about why your research matters is one good way of keeping yourself honest, and your research useful and relevant, not taking off on its own, just because you got started on it. At first, others may often be less interested than you are, in the specific issues and facts you have studied in detail; they will likely want to know, bluntly, "So what?" Therefore, it's a good practice to ask yourself that question, now and then, as you are working and writing, and to give your own answers to it. What does it tell us, that we didn't know before? What decision or policy or action is illuminated by it? What should anyone do on the basis of it? These are fair questions, for all of us.

At some point, we will likely have to discuss in detail our findings; and as we've discussed before, and will reiterate below, be transparent about the process through which we came to our conclusions. Once our audience sees that our action research may have some relevance and value to them, then, at that point, they may be more ready to hear some of the details of the "story" of our action research project—the processes that led to the results.

An important part of any scientist's openness to change, and our respect for collaboration and for correction by our colleagues, lies in our willingness to be clear about how we got to the conclusions we have reached. We should try to include some of this in all our research writing. We are not simply giving end-results or telling final conclusions. We are giving our readers a picture of a process, an inquiry, investigating issues and seeking for conditional truths, which we can use and offer to others as useful. That means our conclusions are only as good as our process, our evidence, the ways we formulate and reason about their interconnections. We want others to tell us how they got to their conclusions, after all; traditional research forms often do this in very irritating and stereotyped ways, which often mask the reality they describe, as much or more than they clarify it. Instead of telling something of the actual process of inquiry, standard journal articles, for example, tend to report data in a retrospective rhetoric of conclusions—terse, quantitative tables, together with mention of statistical tests used in assessing them, the "confidence levels" or certain measures of reliability, and perhaps the "hypotheses confirmed" or "not supported." A brief "Discussion" section may tell something, minimally, of what all this may mean, and an even briefer "Conclusions" section will typically re-state what was already said, in summary form. It is all artificial, backward-looking, cast in a pseudo-objective mode that is designed to look concise, precise, and rigorous. These are the images of "science" as the traditional view has it, and that we have been taught by most textbooks. But there are other ways to do it.

In community-related action research, it often makes sense to start where the research itself started—with the reasons for wanting to do it at all. This may be an interest of the community board, for example, in knowing about what the agency is doing, or how well it is doing it. It may be a personal interest of the researcher. It may be an outside agency's demands, which start the research, but hopefully, not the only reason for doing it. Then, we can tell about important decisions that were made as the study went along—what scope and coverage it should have, how much money and time there is available to do it, what its main purposes are to be, who is to do it, using what methods, who else is to be involved, and so on.

Describing major changes of direction as the research progressed can be quite important, to help our readers understand the process and its results. It can also be helpful to readers if we describe whom we've talked to, what kinds of documents were analyzed, what revisions and critiques were done within the organization, what changes happened in the organization as we went through the study, because of things learned in the process. Such changes are sometimes the most significant consequences of an action research project. We should be sure to discuss our main ways of analyzing the data—not just the technical, statistical methods—but our ways of thinking about the issues. These can be sometimes be communicated concisely, with practice, or as I will discuss next, they can sometimes be told in terms of vivid, tangible storytelling. So, for example, there are ways of including in our report much of the "raw data," in the form of direct quotations from a number of interviewees. Specific quotations, or detailed stories of what was observed or learned, can give readers a chance to check our inferences from those data, and to agree or disagree with our conclusions, from their own analyses of the evidence we've presented, along with how and why we interpreted the evidence the way we have.

How far to go in filling out your description of the actual process of our research is a matter of judgment, to be made in light of our study's purposes, the audiences we intend it for, and the space and time available in writing it up. But the thrust of our efforts should be toward telling a full, natural, honest story of what actually happened, leaving out what is merely incidental or of passing interest, and focusing on the main points of the whole thing, along with some well-chosen specific details and illustrations. The purpose is to let our readers come to understand how we got there, as well as where we "ended up." That is a better way of being transparent, and it is more critical than assuming a pretense of "objectivity" by merely repeating the proper technical mumbo-jumbo for the research discipline we may want to impress.

These are just some of the issues involved in writing about action research. Each of us will have many ideas of our own about the subject, things that have worked for us. Also, each of us may have identified "blocks," or problems, that arise for us repeatedly, when starting to do writing about action research projects. Next, I will discuss the importance of "sharing stories" as well as the importance of "writing in our own voice," along with some further, potentially helpful writing strategies.

Putting ourselves at the heart of telling the story of our action-inquiry, in our own voice

Now, I aim to discuss further a few principles of good communication in doing transformative action research, most of which have been previously, even if only briefly, discussed in this book. First, when writing about an action-inquiry in which we have been engaged it is *important for us to put ourselves at the heart of the "story" of the action-inquiry about which we are writing.* This means:

1. sharing with our readers (or listeners) the thinking behind the decisions we make at various steps along the way when doing the action research, in order to be transparent to others and engage the readers, or listeners, in our thought processes during the inquiry; this includes writing to convey not just generalizations and abstract concepts by themselves, but also to connect ideas and conclusions with a variety of specific examples. This means using storytelling, case studies, and detailed illustrations.
2. writing in our own voice and from our own perspective.

Telling stories, connecting generalizations with examples

I'd like to consider several approaches: 1) being a "tour guide"; 2) going beyond abstractions to well-illustrated, nuances about the complexities of emerging knowledge; and 3) storytelling and painting a picture to make "soft" data "hard."

Being a "tour guide"

We can aim to act something like "tour guides" on a bus traveling through a landscape, well-known to us, but unfamiliar to the tourists on the bus. In looking out the window of the bus (that is, in looking at the action research we have done and what we have learned and/or are still doing and learning about), we should point out specific details of the landscape—both themes in the landscape such as common rock formations and colors, but also variations, such as an unusual cluster of vegetation on an otherwise arid landscape. As we do this, we should try to add further anecdotes and stories that reveal interesting connections. How does this landscape compare with other landscapes? Why is it different and how did it come to be different? What does it feel like when we get out and walk through the landscape? Why is this important to us or interesting? Further, we might share a story someone told us about the history of what has gone on among the rock formations, perhaps in the 1930s, Hollywood made Western movies with "shoot-outs" between the "good guys" and the "bad guys" hiding behind these boulders. Metaphorically speaking, such questions and added comments are quite relevant when discussing our research. In literal terms, we should aim to paint a vivid picture of the various circumstances surrounding our action-inquiry.

For example, as discussed earlier, when I was involved in the assessment of elder needs for a major city's redevelopment agency, I was told not to take time to assess their needs for housing because those needs had already been met. Then I later found out that housing was a huge, unmet need. This was not only "surprising" and "noteworthy" information, I also found myself feeling upset. Why? Because the redevelopment agency staff were perhaps being negligent, oblivious to the inadequacy of the millions of dollars they had obtained for building "low income" housing that had failed to become homes for the elders most in need? Or perhaps the agency staff had become aware of this failure and wanted to cover it up? In either case, these upsetting possibilities were part of the "story" for me, and not just the "research methods," and a reminder that one always needs to be open to modifying one's initial research questions. The added part of the story seemed to be also that public agencies sometimes fail to see to it that resources that are intended for those most in need fulfill their intended purpose. If I were writing about this inquiry, this would be part of my "tour guide's" commentary on the "landscape" of that story of action-and-inquiry.

Going beyond abstractions to well-illustrated nuances about the complexities of emerging knowledge

Providing tangible, illustrative details of our general findings and insights when doing action research is exceedingly important in adequately conveying the subtleties and nuances of any generalizations or themes that are at the heart of our conclusions. In Chapters 3 and 6, I discussed Blumer's notion of "sensitizing concepts," where concepts are not vague abstractions, but also richly illustrated with and connected to a variety of relevant examples (Blumer, 1969). Stories, case studies, and detailed examples are all critical in communicating what we know and what we have learned through our action-inquiries. This is also important, because as the Dreyfus brothers have articulated in their theory of knowledge development, expert knowledge, at the highest levels, and the most profound depths, is best conveyed not just by rules, techniques, and concepts, but also by sharing one's reservoir of experience. This involves telling and sharing stories along with commentaries and analyses of what those stories suggest, that is, with the insights one can gain from those stories (Dreyfus & Dreyfus, 1985).

That is, expert knowledge must draw on extensive experience, which cannot be boiled down to or substituted by rules or algorithms no matter how well developed. In writing about our research, it can be extremely important to include lots of stories and examples to illustrate the details and complexities of our insights and conclusions. The importance of this is often overlooked. Unfortunately, many experts who write books and conduct training sessions instruct others in the basic concepts, principles, and techniques that they, the very wise and experienced experts understand because they have learned them over many years through extensive trial and error, as well as through systematic inquiry, and by experiencing some quite varied circumstances and situations. However, less expert people cannot begin to appreciate the subtleties of expert knowledge, nor the further inquiry and experience necessary to develop that level of knowledge, without the benefit of more specific illustrations.

I refer everyone to an excellent article written by the late Professor Emeritus of Philosophy, UC Berkeley, Hubert Dreyfus, with his brother Stuart (who was a Professor of Engineering there): "From Socrates to Expert Systems: The Limits and Dangers of Calculative Rationality" (Dreyfus & Dreyfus, 1985). I've been handing out a shorter version of this article for many, many years at WISR. I sat in on some of Hugh Dreyfus' lectures at UC Berkeley when I was doing research on outstanding teachers. Dreyfus was highly regarded by his students, and I had the pleasure of interviewing him. This online article and the old article with the faded copier image that I've been handing out is about "expert knowledge" and potentially applicable to any field we might imagine—be it playing chess, flying airplanes, teaching in alternative schools, practicing as a therapist, or working as an auto mechanic. The two brothers wrote an earlier article for the Air Force on the response of pilots of differing levels of expertise and experience to emergency/crisis/novel situations. Arguably, the expert knowledge that is developed in realms involving work with human beings is every bit as complex, if not more so, than playing chess or flying a plane.

It seems that those who are most expert have a knowledge foundation based on extensive experience, and also on experience that is carefully, intently, and critically reflected upon. A main insight of the Dreyfus brothers about the highest levels of expert knowledge is that, beyond an understanding of general principles, having extensive experience is essential. The expertise growing out of that experience can't simply be boiled down to or replaced by principles or algorithms, alone. Certainly, well-developed principles and complex algorithms are better than the "novice" level of expertise which usually employs a limited, "cookbook" approach of learning a few simple, introductory techniques or rules. What we can learn from the Dreyfus brothers explains something else that I have long observed—that those trained by experts are very, very rarely even close to being as skilled and expert as the experts who have trained them. Why? For one thing, "experts" don't go "though a training program and then suddenly become experts."

Experts become expert because of their extensive experience, and that experience unfolds over time, usually also drawing on some intangible, though not unattainable, qualities of creative thinking, imagination, conviction, dedication, critical-mindedness, willingness to explore and experiment, curiosity, openness to change, tolerance for ambiguity, and much more. Indeed, these are qualities and processes that I have come to appreciate and have tried to nurture in myself and others, as essential to what I'm calling "transformative action-inquiry."

Certainly, some who go to the trainings conducted by experts already possess, or are easily able to further develop, some of the expert's knowledge and qualities. At the very least, most will have a predisposition to be able to develop such expert qualities, but the presentations and discussions in even a whole series of "training sessions" seldom have sufficient emphasis *on the process by which the presenter(s) developed the insights and skills "presented."* All too seldom do the trainees gain an appreciation for the *processes* through which, over time, knowledge and skills are refined and more deeply developed, as one gains the years of necessary experience.

The best trainings are probably "apprenticeships" or "internships" where experts provide trainees/learners/apprentices with opportunities to *learn with them*, with opportunities to experience on their own, as well as to observe the experts, and quite importantly also, opportunities to "scratch their heads" with the expert and talk and think out loud about "problems." Notice that this is different from the expert simply "telling" the apprentice what they should learn in the situation. Not that there is anything wrong with some such instruction, "notice this, learn from that, see how this principle or circumstance played out here." That can be valuable, but it is very, very insufficient. *It is ideal for the apprentice to be with the expert while the expert continues to be engaged in their process of becoming more expert. The expert still scratches their head, runs up against problems, sometimes feels undecided, and the apprenticed learner sees how the process of fine-tuning and creating knowledge and expertise is always ongoing.*

Consequently, when the expert is writing about what they know, they have some special challenges in communicating their knowledge, since they are not working "side by side" with the people to whom they are trying to communicate. Furthermore, if you have done some action research project, you are at the very least in the process of becoming an expert, and very likely may have the beginnings (or more!) of some expert knowledge on the topic or situation in which you have been engaged. This is yet another reason, beyond transparency alone, that you should aim to share with your readers (or listeners) some sense of the process by which you have come to your insights. You should try to do so not just by providing general conclusions or insights, but also by illustrating the ideas with specific examples or at least some tangible explanatory details. At the higher levels of expert knowledge, people come to appreciate the importance of variation—of exceptions to the rules, of situational and contextual differences, and of nuances and subtleties that cannot be so easily boiled down to a short list of definitive concepts and assertions.

Storytelling and painting a picture to make "soft" data "hard"

As noted in Chapter 7, discussing how we judge and evaluate evidence involves more than looking for "hard data" and rejecting or questioning "soft data."

Potentially all data can be valuable, and all data can be potentially misleading, if we do not critically evaluate our data, and try to build a meaningful and coherent picture that "makes sense." In a previously discussed example, in solving a murder case, a detective may do a lab analysis of the kind of bullet found in a body and search for the gun from which it was fired. This seems like it is fairly "objective" or quantitative data. But usually without some other data, like a suspect being observed shooting the gun or at least seen running from the house soon after the murder time—things that might be considered "subjective" or "soft" data; so, depending on the circumstances and credibility of the observation, it's hard to make even a tentative, conclusion or "case." Even finding a DNA sample on the victim's body may only "prove" that the suspect was in contact with the victim, maybe even in a fight with the victim. Still, without additional, "confirming" evidence of another sort (oftentimes "soft" data, like the suspect's motive, and added observations) it will be hard to make a case "beyond a reasonable doubt." Specific details are important to "paint a picture" of what happened, and even so, people may disagree on what the picture "means."

Both so-called "hard" and "soft" data can be used to corroborate or support one another, or to call one another into question. Sometimes, one might feel the soft data is more important even though the "hard data" may appear to be unambiguous. To take a different example, in studying the complexities of mind-body health, it may be unambiguous that my blood looks like "healthy" blood, with an active immune system. "Other things being equal" that may bode well for my health, but it doesn't guarantee that I'm "really" going to be more resistant to an infection than someone with "less healthy" blood indicators. The realities of the health of my immune system, physically, and perhaps in terms of extremely difficult to assess mind-body-spirit conditions, or other unknown relevant physical conditions, are likely much more complex. Painting an illuminating and "accurate" picture of my health, or anyone's health, involves using *a lot* of specific details, and requires our trying to understand the interrelationships of a whole host of considerations.

In summary, as we write about our research findings, we should try to engage our readers, or listeners, in *being with us* as we think about and wrestle with the insights we have come to through our experience, that is, through our action research. To best do this, we need to include many examples and stories, and to invite our readers and listeners to be engaged with us, in the process of becoming more expert with an appreciation of specific details and nuances among varying situations and contexts, beyond the mere assertion of "general findings."

Writing in your own voice

(Revised and updated from an earlier article written by Dr. Cynthia Lawrence.)
In communicating what we have learned from our inquiries, as well as about our purposes in pursuing our action-inquiries, it is important that we learn to write in our own voice. Certainly, some peer-reviewed journals require that we not write in our own voice, as if writing in our own voice proves that we are biased, and not

doing so is not then evidence of careful inquiry, which many believe requires an attitude of detachment. However, writing in a detached tone does not prove that one has been rigorous, and by writing in one's own voice, one may more easily be transparent about the strengths, and the limitations, of one's approach to the inquiry, thereby allowing the reader to critique the methods and evidence of that inquiry. So, at WISR, and when doing transformative action research, we advocate learning how to write in one's own voice. If necessary, you can later rewrite your article or book in a different voice if that is absolutely required by someplace where you have chosen to publish.

Here's what Dr. Cynthia Lawrence, a WISR faculty member and a long-time faculty member at University of California San Diego in Teacher Education had to say to WISR students about "writing in your own voice." These words of guidance were also based on her many years of experience as a schoolteacher focusing on multicultural inclusiveness and language skill development. [The rest of this section has been quoted from previous unpublished writing and seminar presentations made by Dr. Lawrence, with light editing, and with her permission].

I started the seminar with a task that asked the group to punctuate this sentence: "Woman without her man is nothing." As there were many feminist women in attendance, the sentence was quickly punctuated, "Woman; without her, man is nothing."

I have been known to say that the mechanics of language are the least important aspect of writing, and I still say that. Although, I have just shown that punctuation can change the meaning and the intent of what the writer has to say. However, it is a greater concern that mechanics—punctuation, grammar, spelling and so on, not stop writing from happening.

I have also been known to say that a good editor can fix written work, and that the creator of the writing needs to worry about content more than form. However, I have recently had an example of a graduate student who turned her work over to an editor who completely removed her "voice"—what she wanted to say—in a way that removed what was emotionally poignant and crucially appropriate to the subject matter of which she spoke.

I will not stop giving the advice I have given about mechanics or the editing process, but I will temper it with the reality that one must be diligent about being heard. As someone once said, "No one can express your ideas as well as you can." So, even the best editor is only good if they leave your voice clearly heard.

We, at WISR, accept and legitimate, validate and honor your subjective voice. We expect that you write, not to show you're right but to show that you have a legitimate position. The knowledge you bring to the subject of discussion is valuable and comes from a variety of sources, some of which you might not even be aware of. Knowledge comes from life experience, from interactions with co-workers, from media (both mainstream and alternative), and from the Internet and beyond.

Writing is …

1. The preservation of thought.
   a. By simply writing down ideas, and not trusting memory, one can record what is to be said and how it would be best stated. Once recorded, ideas can be read and finessed to make your point exactly the way you wish to make it.
   b. The way to record field notes, ethnographies, theories, and concepts. Everyone finds their own way to reflect on their ethnographic experience in the field. What comes out of interviews may be more than words or may be words that are expressed in ways different from your experience. Writing about your field experience while recording field notes, enriches the content and results of your action research. It is also important to record notes before they get "cold."
2. The clarification of thought.
   a. Thoughts are often unfinished or not clearly stated. Once written, thoughts can be read for clarity, rearranged to provide an inviting flow of ideas, and sequenced in ways that the reader can follow easily.
3. The encouragement of communication with others
   a. Your thoughts spark thoughts in others. I often read someone else's work to get inspiration for my own writing. Once our thoughts are written down, others can respond to what we've said, in cooperative and synergistic ways.
4. The format for dissemination
   a. In order for our work, which is the proof of our knowledge—often experiential and unique—to be used collaboratively, it must be in written form. Having your writing published is reinforcing in many ways. However, even if the work is not formally published, it can still add to the body of knowledge of social change.
5. The content that adds to society's body of knowledge
   a. Action research is one of the ways to give voice to the marginalized part of our society, which is often overlooked. Although writing has been used as a standard by which to judge society's level of civilization, I am not suggesting that none of us have to prove our self-worth by becoming expert writers. I am, however, suggesting that we use writing to add to what is being said about the segments of our society left out of, and misrepresented in, the "body of knowledge" that is incomplete without us.
6. The proof of what one learns.
   a. For WISR, your writing is the organized and thoughtful product of your knowledge-building. Most universities require written work. The

difference here is that WISR wants to hear your thoughts and your theories, along with information you've gathered through action research, synthesized with readings and other information-gathering activities.

7. The validation of personal knowledge.

   a. Once something is committed to paper in written form, it can be read and responded to. Readers give much-needed validation of our knowledge-building process.

8. The commitment to paper – ideas, values, philosophy.

   a. I hear that some people really enjoy the process of writing. Personally, I tend to procrastinate and struggle to meet deadlines when I have a writing project. I don't find writing easy. One of the things I think needs to be changed about writing is the choice to write in ways that are comfortable and expressive. Others do judge our writing, and indirectly we are judged too. When expressing ideas and values, one is taking a chance on being rejected. Using certain terms that are value-laden allows others to categorize us in sometimes inappropriate and erroneous ways. It is a commitment, and not an easy process.

In order to maintain the integrity of your message, you must write in your own voice. So, what is one's own voice? It is the voice that allows you to express your own values, philosophies, social theories, cultural experience, political position, and passions and more. Both John (Bilorusky) and I have experienced reading a paper without the name of the writer and knowing exactly who wrote the paper. That is to say that if you truly write in your own voice, your signature might not even need to be there for readers to know your writing. Still, it is a good idea to put your name on your writing, to own your writing. Therefore, what you write must be something you are willing to own and even be proud of.

Before I go further, I need to blast all those elementary and secondary teachers of English who blocked your writing growth rather than having expanded it. I have seen students express that the red pen on their papers made them think that the teacher had made the student's writing bleed. Their souls might have bled from the attack on their sincere attempt to put their thoughts down on paper. Yes, a teacher's responsibility is to "correct" writing, but that correction of mechanics must be separated from the content and from the expression of thought. Although there must be a standard form that allows us some universal ability to read one another's work, the learning of that standard can, and should, be done during another part of the learning process.

When I was teaching young writers in fifth grade classroom, I set up editing centers. A small group of learners would work with me to become experts in some area of written mechanic—spelling, punctuation, syntax and so on. The other children would take their work to the experts for editing. Eventually, all children were experts in all areas, and writing mechanics were checked in a non-threatening way. Writing that was put on display, or sent home or sent out of the classroom, was considered "published." All writing had to be edited before it could be published.

Unfortunately, all of us did not receive such an unthreatening approach, nor even a clear understanding of the mechanics of writing. Nor were we taught how to find our voice and express ourselves. Therefore, it may be hard to trust our voice, our style, our emotional self, our values, our intellect, and more.

These thoughts, drawn from a previous seminar, do not express all the information and inspiration of that seminar. You are only hearing my voice. The richness of the other voices is missing. But I have recorded some of the ideas from the seminar. As I said, write it down!

As a follow-up I've also listened to the recording of a workshop done by John (Bilorusky) and Terry (Lunsford). I listened to the recording of the workshop that I was not able to attend. I used the information from the recording and have then added my own, further ideas, structure, and personal experiences about writing, which I would like to share and highlight here, as things to keep in mind when writing.

The following is a structuring of key points to keep in mind—that came from the writing workshop:

1. Kinds of Writing (or Purpose of Writing):
   - writing language is the preservation of thoughts.
   - writing is a form of communication and sharing of thoughts.
   - academic writing—for the publication of one's position.
   - recreational writing—where one enjoys flow of thoughts and the expectation of ideas yet to be revealed also, stream of consciousness—journals and diaries writing that is often free from critique and evaluation.
   - knowledge of appropriate writing form, keeping one's audience(s) in mind.

2. Steps to Writing:
   - save the "pearl" (the main essence of your point or thought).
   - take notes—record ideas, as a routine practice and habit to develop.
   - extensive vocabulary—growth exercises to improve the variety of words used, to convey nuances, without trying to sound "expert" or esoteric.
   - ideas, experiences, and background reading—all contribute to the content of writing.
   - mechanics—grammar, punctuation, structure, etc.—are important but not the first things to address.
   - models of writing—one can use of literature to learn written models of writing; one can also learn how to write from how we talk.
   - brainstorming ideas with others can contribute to writing.

- pattern building orally with clarification of thought (through our response) is another model for how we can write.
- awareness of talking to different issues and in different roles—such awareness can help us to write from "different angles."
- oral skills development is important—including in improving grammar and mechanics, as well as the organization of thought, especially if we do so with an awareness of the transfer to of what we do well orally to what we can do in writing.
- pre-writing—making lists or outlines and categorizing and organizing thoughts—is important.
- preparing a draft and sharing it, and then getting feedback, corrections, and changes, can be very valuable, really critical.
- the "read-around" can provide feedback, informal evaluation, and sharing of our writing efforts with peers, advisors, and friends.

3. Commitment to Writing:
    - writing holds one accountable, and writing widens one's audience.
    - writing may create authority; writing can preserve a sense of success—writing can help us to achieve goals and objectives.
    - writing becomes public—this should be an eventual goal, even if sharing only with one or two others.
    - writing always has purpose—writing must preserve "the pearl" the part of what we have to say that is especially valuable, or potentially so, to ourselves and others. In this way, the writer becomes an actor, a doer.

4. Standards of Writing:
    - academic writing can be clear and simple.
    - writing should be analytical, intellectual with ideas clearly explained and well described.
    - broadness of exposure requires some common standards, such as:
        a. writing requires clarity of relationship between points,
        b. writing should highlight important points and supportive evidence.
    - publishing requires specific standards and form, often particular to the requirements of a journal or publisher.

5. What Encourages Writing?
    - Success—is it defined by extrinsic positive evaluations from others, and/or self-satisfaction with what one has written and/or comfort with the process.
    - communication is encouraged by one's goal(s) and audience(s).
    - reduce gap between personal writing and academic writing is quite possible—often, by making formal writing more honest and direct.

- generating your very "pearl," your key idea, and then watching it take shape can be encouraged by making an audio recording of your ideas, and then writing from talk.

6. Ways of Maintaining Meaning ... You can:
    - Often refer to your main point(s), or title.
    - be mindful of writing to your targeted audience(s).
    - write an informal letter to someone about an idea.
    - continually check on the evolving direction of your action-inquiry and focus on points and the relationships between those points and—-for constructive criticism.

By the end of the seminar, there were some important questions left unanswered. Two of them were:

- How can one be comfortable enough to be prolific?
- Does writing flatten expression?

A humorous but sincerely written song, by some of us here at WISR, has the following refrain for the chorus: "Write, Write, Write!" It's not so easy to do, and the process involves periods of being inhibited, and other periods of being quite self-aware and conscious of our purposes and audiences. Nevertheless, writing is very important and can be used to educate others, to work for social change or organizational improvements, or, "just" and quite importantly, contribute to our own action-inquiry and the action-inquiry of others. So, all together now ...

"Let's write, write, write!!"

9

ISSUES AND STRATEGIES OF QUANTITATIVE ANALYSIS

Introduction

Clearly, the transformative approach to action-inquiry emphasizes qualitative research more than quantitative and statistical research. It's not that numbers, and counting things, don't matter. They do. However, it's best to think of them as observations, or inferences about observations, as *one* important piece, or pieces, either of evidence or assessments of evidence. *All too often numbers stop inquiry, rather than promote inquiry. Because of their seemingly definitive quality, numbers can sound like "answers," rather than additional, and sometimes valuable, information. Without critically examining what the numbers mean in light of our qualitative understanding of what the numbers are about, using numbers alone, by themselves, may oftentimes be misleading.*

Inquiry may be stopped, when numbers are used simply to "prove" or "disprove" hypotheses, oftentimes by stating the degree to which a statistical procedure has "told us" to be confident in the likelihood of our conclusion being correct. This may lead us away from studying further the variations on the result and the exceptions. However, by studying variations and exceptions more closely, we may gain not only important insights about things that are unusual, but also very often, a deeper understanding about the subtle dynamics underlying what is the most common theme or tendency. Unfortunately, instead, some researchers decide pretty much once and for all, what specific quantitative indicators we should look at in assessing what are oftentimes very complex dynamics that are still not yet fully understood. Consequently, many people settle on the agreed-on quantitative measures, and "that's that." Economic well-being then becomes defined in terms of a few things such as the Dow Jones Industrial Average (only about the stock market), the Gross National Product, or the unemployment rate (which fails to count the chronically unemployed and underemployed).

Quite relevant to these reflections on the limitations of quantitative measures is the extremely eloquent speech made by Robert F. Kennedy on March 18, 1968, just several months before he was assassinated:

> Too much and for too long, we seemed to have surrendered personal excellence and community values in the mere accumulation of material things. Our Gross National Product, now, is over $800 billion dollars a year, but that Gross National Product—if we judge the United States of America by that – that Gross National Product counts air pollution and cigarette advertising, and ambulances to clear our highways of carnage. It counts special locks for our doors and the jails for the people who break them. It counts the destruction of the redwood and the loss of our natural wonder in chaotic sprawl. It counts napalm and counts nuclear warheads and armored cars for the police to fight the riots in our cities. It counts Whitman's rifle and Speck's knife, and the television programs which glorify violence in order to sell toys to our children. Yet the gross national product does not allow for the health of our children, the quality of their education or the joy of their play. It does not include the beauty of our poetry or the strength of our marriages, the intelligence of our public debate or the integrity of our public officials. It measures neither our wit nor our courage, neither our wisdom nor our learning, neither our compassion nor our devotion to our country, it measures everything in short, except that which makes life worthwhile. And it can tell us everything about America except why we are proud that we are Americans. (Taylor, 1970)

What can we do about this?

Demystifying statistics and quantitative vs. qualitative approaches to weighing evidence

Throughout this chapter, I'd like for us to keep in mind that our decisions are always made by us, not by numbers, for we always choose how to use numbers, and what meaning and importance to give to numbers. In order to discuss better the importance of qualitatively understanding quantitative analyses, I wish to describe, and review, widely practiced quantitative approaches, discuss the reasoning and assumptions behind these approaches, and note their uses and limitations.

Generally speaking, there are two types of uses of "statistics"—

1. A numerical "fact"—in this sense, "statistics" involves counting things (e.g., she has five brothers and sisters) or using some standard of "measurement" (e.g., he is six feet tall and has an IQ of 105). This is sometimes referred to as descriptive statistics.
2. A field of study, which uses mathematical methods to help people to make sense out of large, and/or complicated, masses of information. In this sense, statistical techniques are used both to describe groups of people, types of

programs and situations, and the like, and also to draw inferences, or make indirect conclusions, or "calculated" judgments about similarities, differences, and relationships between two or more groups of people, groups of events and circumstances, or types of programs, for example. This is usually called inferential statistics.

Inferential statistics is used to study possible causal connections between two or more factors or variables. The following is a brief overview of one main approach to inferential statistics, using statistics to make inferences about whether there is a strong relationship between variables that may suggest that one factor *might* cause a type of outcome.

Estimating the likelihood that a causal connection might exist—statistical tests of "significance"—uses and limitations

Weighing and judging a variety of pieces of evidence is often part of a process of deciding between two or more alternative courses of action. This judgment process is much more complicated and involved than the hypothesis-testing approach commonly used in conventional research; however, it is informative for us to look at and understand the reasoning behind the more simplified hypothesis-testing approach.

Using that approach, the researcher begins with a hypothesis, such as: "Thirty-second public service announcements on local TV stations can be used effectively to educate the public about various community health problems." The researcher then makes an initial hypothesis that the statement is false, or incorrect, unless they can marshal "sufficient" convincing evidence to the contrary. That is, researchers tend to take the conservative position of assuming that their hypothesis about a relationship between two factors or "variables" is false, until they have significant evidence contradicting the falsehood of their hypothesis. So, they see if they are able to disprove that the relationship does not exist.

Without going into all the computational and mathematical details here, let's just say that there are statistical procedures, agreed upon by mathematicians and by social and natural scientists who use those procedures, for crunching and interpreting the numbers they get. Those who are interested in learning more can find many very good explanations of the details online and in textbooks and just to get you started there are three, different web links that may be instructive (Nigam, 2018; Khan Academy, n.d.; Gallo, 2016).[1]

Here, I wish to help you to understand only the *thinking* behind *tests of statistical significance when one wants to estimate* the likelihood of a relationship. Consider the above mentioned, hypothetical example of the question, as to whether Public Service Announcements (PSAs) on TV are the better strategy for educating people on matters of health.

- First, if we believe that they likely may be educational, we will hypothesize the *opposite*. We will state, "PSAs are *not* effective in educating people on health issues."
- Second, if doing a "controlled laboratory experiment," we will *test* the hypothesis by putting together *two samples*. One sample will include people who see a certain number of PSAs on some matter of public health—perhaps the importance of not drinking beverages that contain a lot of added sugar. The other sample of people will not be exposed to the PSA messages. Further, we will want to make sure that each sample is roughly comparable, or similar, to one another. We don't want the samples to be different in ways that we think might matter—such as the amount of college education, their occupations, income levels, gender, racial and cultural identification, exercise routines, or current dietary practices. So, the researcher will take one group of people, and *from that group randomly assign* one subgroup to watch some PSAs, while the other group does not. A limitation is that the "overall group" that the researcher starts with might not be "typical" of the *diversity* of the whole population to which the researcher wants to generalize their findings. For example, such studies often use college students because researchers can get them to participate, but if so, the results of these studies might not be generalizable, or applicable, to people who are different from college students in important ways that might matter, in terms of the research hypothesis. For example, the general population might be older, less educated, less affluent, or different in ways we can't easily anticipate or identify.
- Another option, if the researcher is studying people's behavior in the real world, is to study the "sugary beverage consumption behavior" among two large samples of people in the general population. Then, they must "statistically" examine how naturally occurring subgroups are different (or not) in their soft drink consumption in relation to the frequency of having seen such PSAs. For example, among people of a certain age group, or ethnic group, or income group, or some other grouping, does sugar drink consumption go down, or not, for those people who see a lot of PSAs about this topic.
- Further, the researchers must figure out how to accurately measure people's attitudes, or ideally, their behavior, about drinking sugary beverages. How often do they drink sugary beverages? They must assume that people's self-reports are accurate or try to double check this by carefully interviewing the participants (and such careful interviews then move us into the domain of using at least some qualitative methods). With laboratory studies, the researchers can show those in the experimental group a certain number of PSAs and none to the control group. With real world research, the researchers must interview everyone about how often they see such PSAs, and hope that people provide them with relatively accurate information about what they recall.
- In the case of a controlled laboratory experiment, it is necessary to "test" people before and after the study. For people in each group, at the beginning of the study, how many people, for example, report drinking one glass, 2

glasses, and maybe as many as 20 glasses of sugar beverages each week. Of course, as noted above, people may not recall accurately, or they may report what they "think" we want to "hear." This is a problem of accurate or valid measurement of their behavior. All research, quantitative and qualitative, and research which uses both approaches, has to *assess as best as possible the validity of the evidence, of the resulting "measurements."*

An inherent challenge, in both real world and "laboratory" settings is that researchers can never "account for" all other variables. There may be important circumstances or personal characteristics that affect how often people drink sugary beverages that will make it difficult for the researchers to "isolate" the impact of PSAs on behavior. They can try to think of all the relevant variables but doing this usually requires that we do extensive *qualitative research, using in-depth interviews and observations.*

Let's now consider the statistical procedures used in the experimental study, without going into the somewhat different statistical analyses done in the case of the "real world research" since this book does not aim to comprehensively address the whole range of statistical methods:

- For the experimental study, the numerical findings about sugary beverage consumption of four groups will be statistically analyzed by considering the results for four groups:
    a. for the control group (those not seeing PSAs) with two results, one for the beginning of the study and another result later at the end of the study (even though they aren't shown any PSAs); and
    b. for the "experimental group" (those seeing PSAs), two results also, "before" and "after" (seeing the PSAs). The results are presented in what mathematicians call probability distributions. These distributions result from numbers (number of drinks of sugary beverage consumed) showing the percentage of people in each sample, before and after the intervention with PSAs who drink the different amounts of sugary beverages.

- Let's look at how this might be graphed:
    a. In this hypothetical example (see the made-up, illustrative graph below, Figure 9.1), I've drawn four lines. The dotted line depicts the experimental group "before" and the black dashed line is for the control group "before." The gray dashed line is the control group "after," and the black line represents the experimental group "after" having seen the PSAs.
    b. Notice that the dotted and gray dashed lines, while not identical, do look a bit like each other. If so, our samples start off "about the same" and using random sampling does increase the likelihood that the two groups will start off with people with similar sugary beverage consumption—about

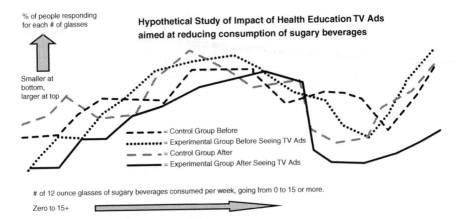

FIGURE 9.1 Four graphs showing the percent of people in each of four hypothetical groups consuming different amounts of sugary beverages each week.

the same percentages of each group drinking very little, similar numbers drinking moderate amounts, and about the same percentage in both groups drinking a lot. Depending on how large our sample size is the mathematical computation may say that they are "close enough." It seems that there are a moderate number of people represented on the left side of the graph who consume little or few sugary beverages, then there is a bit of a "hump" in the middle suggesting that a fair number of people drink them somewhat regularly, and then there is a large number who may be quite "addicted" or at least who drink a lot each week, maybe two or more glasses per day.

c. The gray dashed line represents the control group which was tested again later but without seeing the PSAs, and in our "make-believe" example, the black dashed line is not too different from the gray dashed line, suggesting that maybe people's reporting is fairly accurate and they do not change their behavior a lot over time. However, the black line represents what was initially the group described by the dotted line, and after seeing the PSAs, this group seems to have changed their behavior somewhat, as is demonstrated by the black line. Specifically, those who consumed little or moderately in the way of sugary beverage didn't change their behavior dramatically after seeing the PSAs, but the black line is much lower at the high end of sugary beverage consumption. Consequently, it appears that those who started off drinking a lot of sugary beverages have now decreased their consumption after seeing the PSAs. It appears that *perhaps the PSAs persuaded those who were consuming the most in sugar beverages to at least moderate the extent of their consumption.*

d. Going from left to right: 0 (zero) sugary beverages consumed each week to perhaps 15 glasses per week. Going from bottom to top: 0%

consuming that number of glasses, to the top with a very high percentage consuming that number of glasses per week,
  e. Looking visually at the hypothetical, illustrative graphs (above), my qualitative assessment, or at least "new hypothesis," would be that such PSAs are best in influencing those who consume a lot of sugary drinks each week, or at least influencing them somewhat.

- However, quantitatively focused researchers would not just "eye ball" the graph, but would rely on their statistical computations to calculate the percentage-likelihood or probability that the changes in the "probability distributions" (that is, the change of the black dashed line to the gray dashed line, in comparison with the change of the dotted line to the solid black line) is due to some factor other than random "chance."
- Those who do quantitative research will usually want there to be at least a 95% (perhaps sometimes 99%, or sometimes 90%) likelihood that the differences are not random "chance." If the difference is computed to be this great, they then conclude that it is statistically significant and then they would disprove the hypothesis that PSAs don't make a difference, and therefore conclude that "PSAs might have an impact in educating people about the health value of limiting the consumption of sugar beverages."

So, there are at least two, different outcomes to weighing this evidence statistically. This strictly quantitative approach "gives us" one of two tentative answers—*there is, or there isn't, a "statistical significance" and therefore the hypothesis is proven or disproven.* Then, in either case, we may follow up and do another quantitative study, either the exact same study, or with slightly different groups of people, slightly different PSAs, or with a different health education topic.

Another approach is to *think qualitatively about what they numbers might* mean. As noted above, if I were looking at these four lines, I would notice the following: 1) quite a few people consume no sugary beverages or very few each week, and at the other "end of the scale" there are a really high number who consume a lot of such beverages. (Again, I don't know if this is true—I'm making this scenario up to demonstrate the *process of inquiry*.) 2) It seems that although the PSAs *might* have a very small impact to discourage many people from consuming as much in the way of sugary beverages, the PSAs are most successful in noticeably discouraging those who consumer a large number of such drinks from being quite so excessive in the consumption.

Having noticed these as *possible* trends or dynamics, and a possible value of the PSAs, if I were doing the research, I'd like to interview people and learn more about what's "behind" their behavior. Specifically, I'd really like to hear from those who saw the PSAs, whether or not they think the PSAs influenced them. If so, how? And why? Such information would be valuable in making a more accurate interpretation of the numbers, and beyond this might give us some important insights into how to better design the PSAs. If we do these sorts of things we are now in the realm of qualitative research and moving toward a transformative approach to action research. Note that one may use a quantitative approach with a qualitative approach, and that the two may work together, in many cases. All too often, researchers will rely only, or primarily, on the quantitative approaches.

Types of errors

Continuing on, thinking about this statistical approach to testing a hypothesis, the researcher takes the view that they can make two possible types of errors in weighing the evidence, *and* that it is possible to quantitatively compute the likelihood of each error. Researchers often use certain accepted, statistical procedures for estimating and comparing each of two types of possible errors, before deciding what action to take on their research results.

It's important to understand conceptually what the two types of errors are, and we may also choose to *qualitatively assess* the likelihood *and also the importance* of each type of error. The first type of possible error would be to incorrectly conclude that the hypothesis is false, when in fact it is correct (i.e., in the above example, one may mistakenly conclude that PSAs might be effectively used for this kind of health education). The second type of possible error would be to incorrectly conclude that the hypothesis is true, when in fact it is false (e.g., it is confirmed that the announcements are not effective when they really might be). Typically, the researcher is "supposed" to err in the direction of concluding that the hypothesis is false, unless there are data that strongly suggest that the error or likelihood of mistakenly concluding that the hypothesis is false when it is not, is very, very low.

That is, with these considerations in mind, the quantitative researcher wants to be able to compute the probability or likelihood of making each of these errors before making a judgment about whether or not to take action based on what they've found. There are well-defined mathematical procedures for doing this that are beyond the scope of this book. For our purposes, I wish to emphasize that while this mathematical convention may be useful as a *starting point* for deciding what to do, *in the final analysis, as inquiring human beings we must decide. The statistical procedures are only tools, and our decisions should ideally include qualitative as well as quantitative evidence, and even perhaps evidence from more than one study or situation.*

As I will discuss later, *the importance of each type of error*—in terms of the impact of an incorrect decision, for better or for worse, in its consequences for individuals and/or the society—is often more critical to consider in action-oriented decision-making than is attention to the likelihood of the error, alone. In this example, the impact of either error would seem not to be catastrophic, but we might well decide that one of the errors has greater consequences than others. If we mistakenly put massive funding and effort into PSAs that we think are effective, but really aren't we've wasted a lot energy and money. If we fail to use PSAs because we think they are ineffective, but really were and could have been, we have lost an important opportunity to improve public health. Which error do you think might be the most impactful?

Unexamined assumptions and over-simplifications and an over-reliance on quantitative analyses

In using statistics, we should not fall into the trap of abdicating our responsibility for, and opportunity to, weigh the evidence from many angles and then make the best judgment that we can, for now. "Judgments" are always qualitative in the final analysis. And, regardless of what we "decide," doing further study and inquiry, often based on further action and newly revised innovations and interventions is always a good idea. I would argue that further study should not be quantitatively oriented, alone.

Let's examine further where the researcher has used a standard, and commonly accepted, statistical procedure to weigh the evidence, and then make a "conclusion" about their hypothesis. Seemingly this method of making judgments is unbiased and objective. Yet, there are significant assumptions and limitations which go into this approach. First, the quantitative measure may be inaccurate, misleading, or irrelevant. In the example under consideration, the questionnaire may not accurately measure people's viewing of PSAs nor their actual behavior in drinking sugary beverages. Also, interpreting the percentage of people answering the questionnaire in a particular way may be ambiguous. For example: is effectiveness with 60 % of the people "twice" as effective as effectiveness with 30%? Or is it "twice" as effective, if the total number of glasses of sugary beverage is cut in half? What if there is only a small margin of difference between what was learned by the 60% and what was learned by the others? What many only changed their behavior for a short period of time? What if the PSAs were very influential with affluent people, but not others, or if they were taken more seriously mostly only by otherwise healthy people who consume a lot of sugar drinks (like I used to!), but then decided to try to become even more healthy by limiting their consumption (as I finally did after many years, of doing otherwise). These are *qualitative questions, and although quantitative information can be used in conjunction with these questions, invariably we cannot rely on the quantitative analyses alone.*

Furthermore, from a mathematical viewpoint, the procedures of statistical analysis make some assumptions. The statistical tests most often used assume that frequency of occurrence of the various values of the what's being measured approximate the "shape" of the famous "bell-shaped" curve—where most people measured (e.g., the amount of sugary beverage consumption by people) are found in the "fat," middle portion of the curve, and very few people, relatively speaking at the two outer "extremes" of the curve. Note that in my hypothetical (but still potentially, believable) example above, the curves were not the usual bell-shaped curve, and indeed, there was an increase near the extreme end of the curve. So, even from a strictly mathematical point of view, the assumptions underlying the statistical calculations do not "fit" the social reality of what is being studied. Such assumptions often are not true, but this is ignored by the statistical methods used to analyze the data. This is just an added problem or limitation that should give us pause about relying too heavily on statistical tests when making our decisions.

In summary, this hypothesis-testing approach is a standardized, but an oversimplified, method of making judgments. Further, it does not consider the human risks and possible benefits involved with each course of action under consideration. Although this approach attempts to estimate the relative likelihood of the two types of possible errors, which can be made in hypothesis-testing, it does not outline a strategy for evaluating the possible human and social consequences of each of the two types of errors. In the example we are considering: What are the costs in terms of time, effort, and money of securing and then producing a public service TV announcement? Might there be a better strategy leading to even more improved public knowledge of community health issues, which could be pursued with about the same expenditure of time, effort, and money? Might we not opt for a more effective strategy even if it involves only "slightly" more time, money, and/or effort?

The value of qualitative approaches to cost-benefit analyses and decision-making

Quite importantly, we now come to yet another, but related, issue. "Slightly" is ultimately a *qualitative* consideration that cannot be quantified. *Very often there is an attempt to put effectiveness, risk, and effort into dollars-and-cents terms, so we can have a neat, and seemingly definitive, cost-benefit equation. But this is an artificial procedure.* Like the oversimplified approach to measuring the "likelihood" of error in the conventional hypothesis-testing approach, quantifying cost-benefit analyses is a contrived procedure, which, by itself, does little to give us the necessary insights into the judgments we are making. These quantitative procedures mislead us into thinking that we have a consistent, objective procedure on which to base our judgments and decisions. In using them, however, we must make many assumptions, which go unexamined and untested by these research procedures. We end up letting these procedures make the judgments for us. Instead, *whenever we are in a position to decide, we should take responsibility for making decisions, using our values and commitments, along with our best judgments in weighing what is often a very complex array of sometimes confusing, contradictory, or at least far from clear cut, evidence.*

The qualitative approach to cost-benefit analysis is to try to collect as much relevant data as possible, especially on the various benefits, costs, and risks associated with each course of action being considered. Then, we must ask such questions as, "What evidence do we have, that points strongly, moderately, or weakly toward various interpretations and conclusions?" For example, some likely benefits of a planned action may be supported only very tentatively and questionably by the data, whereas other advantages, or certain specific risks, may be suggested by extensive and persuasive data. In making judgments about the "meaning" of our data, and about what actions to take, we may have to consider a number of very different pieces of information, pointing in many different directions, and we will undoubtedly use our values in placing more weight on certain pieces of information than on others.

To take another example, the arguments against the use of nuclear power and experimentation with recombinant DNA are based on a technically estimated "likelihood of error" of much less than 5%, or even less than 1/1,000 of 1%. Indeed, advocates of nuclear power and of such biochemical experimentation compute the likelihood of error, or dangers, to be almost zero. Nevertheless, the arguments against these technological practices are based on judgments which give overwhelming importance to the potentially catastrophic consequences to people, and to the larger environment, if we are wrong in assuming with absolute certainty that these courses of action are a 100% safe. No matter how confident we may be, no matter how much statistical evidence we may pile up to support the claim that the likelihood of "accidents" is ever so small, depending on our values and our judgment, we might justifiably say that the consequences are so profound and so irreversible, that, in these cases, the possible impact of the "risk" counts for everything, and considerations about the miniscule "likelihood of error" become completely irrelevant.

With this more qualitative approach to action-inquiry, we can begin to do a "qualitative cost-benefit analysis" by collecting data relevant to costs and risks, and data relevant to benefits. These data are not quantified, but qualitatively stated in human terms, in terms of the practical, ethical, and social consequences over the short term and for the long term. We might choose to include use numbers and statistics, such as economic and financial costs and benefits, as *part* of our decision-making. So considered, even information about financial costs take on a qualitative nature. For example: How much effort do we have to expend to get a $50,000 grant? Could we use our time otherwise? Or, if we already have the money, what are the different ways that we could use the money? *Rather than translating qualitative issues into dollars and cents, we can begin to translate dollars and cents into human terms, and then weigh the evidence. That is, we can make judgments, among possible alternatives, about the information available based on human and social considerations.*

These are just a few of many questions and considerations involved in making decisions, and they will be discussed further in Chapter 13 on ethical considerations.

Rather than "hard" vs. "soft" data, consider different ways of thinking about the world

We can now look at quantitative approaches to research in a new light, as merely one approach to the interpretation of data. Any approach is worthwhile to the extent that it usefully (i.e., accurately and meaningfully) helps us to interpret and understand "reality," to make judgments about that reality and to take action in light of those judgments. Often, however, it is assumed that quantitative approaches are necessarily more accurate because of their numerical precision. It is commonly stated that quantitative approaches use "hard" data and that qualitative approaches use "soft" data. However, *both* types of approaches involve decisions and assumptions about the collection and interpretation of data, and all such decisions should be subject to critical examination. "Data" don't become more "hard" or solid because a number has been assigned to the data. Indeed, all decisions about measurements and the uses of quantitative indicators and results require some judgment. *We—those of us doing the research, engaged in inquiry—inevitably make judgments and decisions about data-gathering and analysis, whether we are doing so qualitatively, quantitatively, or both. In all cases, the solidity and limitations of our process should be transparent and subject to critical examination and evaluation by others!*

Statistical tests, computer simulation models, and all uses of numbers in research are merely quantitative *interpretations* of data. They are valid or invalid, not because of their mathematical precision, but because of the extent to which they accurately and usefully—or inaccurately and not so usefully, as the case may be—enable us to make sense out of data, and to make significant, accurate, and insightful judgments.

As noted above, all statistical tests make assumptions about reality, in collecting the data being fed into the computer or into our calculators. Many statistical tests are quite inconsistent with reality. For example, most statistical tests assume that the variables being studied are smooth, continuous functions. That is, they assume that people and organizations undergo gradual, continuous changes in the areas that we are assessing them. Yet, many social phenomena are characterized by sudden and discontinuous changes of circumstances, or by an abrupt turn of events. The old saying about the "straw that broke the camel's back" is about such unexpected and quite dramatic turns of events. Many processes in our agencies and communities are characterized by such momentous and abrupt occurrences. A relatively new area of mathematics, called "catastrophe or chaos theory" (as well complexity theory) is based on mathematical formulations more in line with such processes than are the statistical tests and procedures typically used in the social sciences, and found in most research texts, be they introductory or advanced.

Physics is often associated with mathematical precision, and yet, developments in physics over the last hundred years have dramatically illustrated how mathematical methods are tools for interpreting data, and as such they can be both useful and misleading. Newton's theories of physics—the theories many of us studied in high school—are based on Euclidian geometry, on mathematical procedures which assume that the shortest distance between two points is a straight line. Einstein brought to our attention that, while Euclidian geometry is useful for understanding many everyday problems, it turns out to be quite limited if we are concerned with questions about the changing nature of the universe. In studying these questions, it turns out that a different kind of geometry is more useful, a geometry which assumes that the space is "curved," and that the shortest distance between two points is not a straight line. In this view of things, we might more usefully think of ourselves as living in a universe, which if flattened out into two dimensions, might be visualized as the surface of a balloon, and the surface of an expanding balloon, at that! So, each point on the surface of the balloon is moving away from one another.

The point of this digression is not to divert our study of educational and community issues to theoretical physics, but to point out that, even in the so-called, very "hard" science of physics, physicists *must decide* which mathematical models and procedures to use. Mathematics is used to help us make sense out of the data, but mathematics cannot make the decisions for us, since we must decide how to use mathematics. That often involves critical thinking, exploratory seeking out of new data, and qualitative, reflective judgments. Physicists inevitably must exercise their judgment, in deciding which mathematical model to use to study any particular domain of reality. So, any application of a mathematical model or procedure is not necessarily valid or useful, even though the mathematics may be "precise." Like the use of any model or method of interpreting data, they are potentially useful, or potentially limiting or misleading, and we must carefully and critically examine them in this light.

Using graphs to think about data

So, I'd like to introduce some statistical and mathematical concepts *and show how these concepts can be illustrated on graphs*. This section will be at bit easier if you have a good understanding of algebra—if you at least are familiar with the idea of plotting data on a sheet of paper with an x-axis running horizontally from left to right and the y-axis as running vertically from top to bottom. Hopefully, those of you who are not so familiar or comfortable with math can follow the gist of what I'm discussing here. Gaining a sense of what the concepts are about, and how to visualize relationships and patters on a graph is much more important than getting lost in the weeds of the mathematical computations.

Normal distribution and "variation"

Most of you may have been exposed at some point to the concept of the "bell shaped curve" or the "normal distribution." In the diagram below, I've shown three different "curves," all of them normal distributions (approximately at least— this is like my drawing on an old-fashioned blackboard, or some newsprint with markers). See the diagram (Figure 9.2) below.

Normal distributions are frequently used because they are a fairly accurate way to depict many (but by no means all!) naturally occurring phenomena. For example, if we study the height of all people in a particular society, or most any *large* group, we will

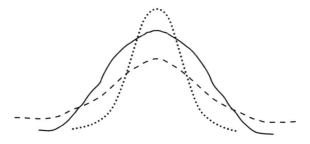

FIGURE 9.2 The shapes of three different normal distributions.

likely find that there are a very large number in the "middle range" of heights, and increasingly smaller numbers as we move toward very tall heights or very short heights. All three drawings above—the black solid, dotted, and dashed—are close approximations of a normal distribution. Notice that the differences are in "how wide" each one is. The more narrow-shaped dotted distribution has what researchers would call "less variation." That is, most of the people (or most of the groups or circumstances if we're assessing those instead of individuals) are close to the middle. If we were measuring the height of people within a group depicted by the dotted line, the vast majority of people would be close to the average height, with extremely few especially tall or especially short people. By contrast the dashed line normal distribution has much more variation, with more people, organizations, or circumstances (depending on what we're measuring) farther toward the extremes, although still most are in the middle area.

Many researchers compute something called *"the standard deviation" to quantify the variation*. If the researchers are studying a very large group, it is often the case that the distribution of values (height, scores, whatever is being measured) approximates the normal distribution. If so, then within one standard deviation above the mean, or midpoint, and going to one standard deviation below the midpoint, 68% of the people (organizations, situations, whatever is being studied) will be in the that "wide, middle portion" of the curve. Hypothetically, if the group's average height is 5 feet, six inches and there is a standard deviation of four inches, then 68% would be between 5 feet, two inches and 5 feet, 10 inches. Statistically, 95% will be within two standard deviations, or in this hypothetical example, 95% would be between 4 feet, 10 inches and 6 feet, 2 inches.

Researchers could study two, different large groups of people to see how the *distribution* of their heights compare, and especially, if there are genetically variables involved, they might find that the distribution for each group is the normal, bell-shaped curve, but that one group is shifted to the right or left of the other group. That is one group is, "on average" taller than the other group. If one were comparing men and women within the same large group, it is likely that this would be their finding. The statistical tests to compare two groups discussed in the previous section would be used to mathematically estimate whether the difference between the two distributions is "likely" a "random" one, or *perhaps* due to some meaningful or interesting cause, such as perhaps genetics in this particular example.

From looking at the three graphs above, we can see that they all have the same midpoint. With a normal distribution, the midpoint is the *median* and the *mean* and the *mode*. This is *not* the case with most other distributions or graphs.

- The "mean" is the way one learns to compute the "average" by adding up the value of all the numbers and dividing by the total number of things added. To keep it simple if we have data for seven people and their "scores" on some test are 2, 2, 2, 3, 8, 8, 11, and if we add the numbers up, we get 35. If we divide 35 by the number of scores/people or 7, we get "5" as the mean or average (even though no one actually scored "5" on the test).

- The "mode" is the most frequently occurring score, and since there are three 2s, 2 is the mode. This hypothetical example is a "bi-modal" distribution where there are two points or values with a high frequency of occurring. In this hypothetical example, there is a second, but smaller "mode" at 8. It seems that on this hypothetical test most everyone scored fairly high or fairly low, with no one in the "middle."
- The "median" is the score that is in the "middle of the list" counting from high to low or low to high (either way), and in this case the number in 4th place, the middle place out of seven numbers, is "3."

In contrast to the very small illustrative sample of seven, above, normal distributions can only result, and even then still, only sometimes, when there is an extremely large sample size, when we are measuring qualities of a much larger number of people, organizations, groups, or circumstances. Further, normal distributions are quite special because the mode, median, and mean are the same! The mode—the most frequently occurring value, whether it is score, income level, height, or whatever we are measuring and studying quantitatively, is also at the midpoint or median of the normal distribution. This is where the "top" of the distribution is. This point is also the computed "average" or "mean."

In Figure 9.2, all three normal distributions have the same mode, median, and mean, but quite different variations or standard deviations. The differences, or variation, in the solid dashed line distribution are much greater than with the solid line one, and this in turn is also greater than the dotted line distribution, where the similarities are greater and the differences less dramatic.

Bi-modal distributions

As mentioned above, bi-modal distributions have two places where a lot of data "cluster." *Figure 9.3 illustrates two different bi-modal distributions*—with the black solid line graph there is about an equal concentration of data (people, organizations, groups, circumstances as assessed by some quality or variable) in two different places (see Figure 9.3). Imagine a class where large numbers students, get either an

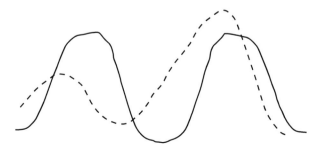

FIGURE 9.3 The shapes of two different bi-modal distributions.

"A" or a "C" on test, or imagine a community where well over a third of the people are employed and making about the same salary, with a similar number of people unemployed and living off of welfare or marginal wages. With the dashed-line graph, there are fewer people on the "left" mode of the distribution and more on the right. This could perhaps depict data in a community where well over half of the people have very good access to health care as measured by the value of health care services they receive, with a significant minority, perhaps 25% or so, who receive only occasional and insufficient health care services.

Normal distributions, and bi-modal distributions, are just two examples of graphs that illustrate how (the frequency with which) within a population or sample certain "characteristics" are "distributed" (among a population or sample of people, groups, or circumstances). That is, for example, in the above examples, how are grades or test scores distributed among students in a particular class, or school? Or how is income distributed among people in a certain community, state or country? One might study, the frequency of acts of violence among the neighborhoods in relation to the average income in that community. In any case, these distributions have a "variable" (such as the test score or grade, the income of individuals, or the average income of different communities, acts of violence, and so forth). Then that is compared in relation to the number of individuals or communities, for example, that are characterized by various "values" of the variables (i.e., different levels of income, or different test scores, etc.). Let's now turn to graphs that illustrate relationships between two variables!

Graphs that describe relationships between two variables

The lines in the graph below (see Figure 9.4) depict several different, important, and fairly common relationships between two variables. *The two, solid black straight lines indicate what is called a linear relationship.* With a linear relationship, a certain increase or decrease in one variable is associated with a proportionate degree of increase or decrease in the other variable. Suppose that one finds that a person's income from age 25 to 65 steadily increases in proportion to their age, perhaps an increase of 5% on average for every year of people's lives. I'm not saying that this is the case, but if it were, it would be a linear relationship with a straight line pointed upward. If the line is pointed at a high angle (as is the case with one of the two solid black lines), it would suggest that income increases dramatically in the group studied as they grow older. If the line were to have a relatively flat, but slightly upward angle (as is the case with the other solid black line), it would suggest instead that income increases as one ages, but not a lot. If the line pointed downward, higher on the left and lower on the right, then, it would suggest that earnings decrease as one ages. One might compare all sorts of variables, such as one's age with one's expressed satisfaction in life. Or the cost of out of pocket health care expenses with one's age. One might compare the success of community agencies as rated by the clients they serve with how long the agencies have been in existence, or with the amount

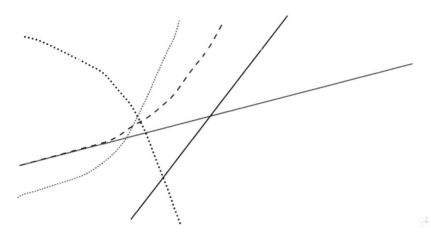

FIGURE 9.4 Five graphs showing significantly different relationships between two variables: Three exponential and two linear.

of funding they receive, or with the years of experience of the leadership team. The numbers and types of variables that could be measured and compared are more than we can even imagine.

Nevertheless, as discussed elsewhere in this chapter and throughout the book, *these quantitatively expressed relationships, even when graphically illustrated do not tell the whole story. We must dig deeper beneath the surface to understand the meaning and significance of the relationships which are only suggested by the numbers and graphic depictions of the numbers.* Without qualitative data and further investigation, including looking at more than just two variables together—since inevitably there are a whole host of relevant variables and considerations—we should not settle on any hard and fast conclusions. *Still, it is fair to say that examining graphs such as these can provide insights and also suggest potentially fruitful directions for next steps in our actions-and-inquiry.*

Looking further at the above graph, there are three other lines drawn, and these are not straight, but curved. After a while, each of them curves rather dramatically, two of them turning upward, and one turning downward. All three of these curved lines are drawn to approximate the way that *an exponential relationship is depicted in a graph*. It is as though the changes indicated by the line start off at a gradual pace, and then "pick up steam" and accelerate. The small-dotted line accelerates even faster and sooner than the dashed line, and the large-dotted line accelerates downward. During the period when I'm drafting this book, the world is in the midst of an evolving pandemic, Covid-19. Early on, and tragically, the number of cases of people being infected with the virus, as well as the number in critical condition and the number who have died, have been accelerating. Most, but disturbingly not all, public leaders are taking steps to try to end this accelerating relationship. They want to slow down the rate at which people are becoming infected with the virus, and of course the rate at which people are dying. They hope to first "flatten" or level out the upward trajectory of the small-dotted and the dashed lines, and then turn them downward, more like the large-dotted line, even if perhaps, sadly, in a less dramatic downward trajectory.

Finally, after a while, many states in the U.S. and many of their residents have been "sheltering at home," and many "non-essential" businesses (including restaurants) are temporarily closed, and as expected, by most indicators the economy is on an accelerating downward trajectory. People are getting laid off work and are unemployed. People are spending less, purchasing only essentials such as food, and pay rent or mortgages if they can afford to do so. Investors in the stock market are worried, and the stock market has been up and down. Certainly, it is debatable as to which economic indicators are truly the most important in terms of human well-being, but by most any indicator, the accelerating downtrend of the large-dotted curved line in the above graph is an apt characterization of our economy.

As the spread and destruction of the virus accelerates exponentially upward (small-dotted or dashed line), the economy is in a free-fall downwards (the large-dotted line).

The discontinuity of "chaos"

The lines that graph relationships between two variables are not always unbroken. So far, we've seen straight lines and curved lines, and they can go up and they can go down. Still, the lines are unbroken, meaning that I could draw the line without ever taking a pen or pencil off the piece of paper. But what if, all of a sudden, after drawing a line that represents the relationships between two variables, I lifted my hand up and "jumped" much higher or lower on the sheet of paper and then proceeded with drawing a line from that new place on the paper. That's what we're looking at in the graph below (see Figure 9.5). There are two lines—a solid line, and dashed line. Let's go back to the current pandemic. Suppose that the first part (on the left) of each of the two lines represents some data prior to the outbreak

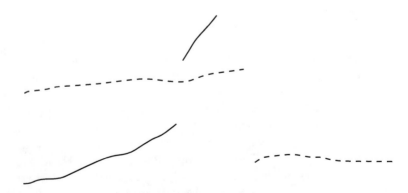

FIGURE 9.5 Two graphs depicting chaos and discontinuity.

of the pandemic. Let's say the solid line represents the number of people infected with the virus. Perhaps, it starts off as a slow, but not really that noticeable, increase. Then, seemingly, "all of a sudden" there is a dramatic increase and the number of cases "jump" almost overnight, and then continue upwards. That's the solid line. Maybe the dashed line is the economy—let's say the average income earned over time by working people in the U.S. It's going along at a steady pace, and then, bam!—overnight the "bottom falls out" and people are laid off work, small business owners have no revenue from customers, and the dashed line jumps downward, and does so "all of a sudden."

These sorts of lines describe the sort of dynamics studied by people who are interested in "chaos theory." It's now easy to see why it has that name. It is the study of how and why, relationships between all sorts of things can dramatically change because of one thing changing, but that one thing matters a lot, and the change is neither smooth, nor gradual, nor usually expected given the way the line "looked" previously. Such lines are "discontinuous," namely they departed dramatically and abruptly from the way they looked before the "chaotic" or "catastrophic" event."

Scatterplots—visualizing a pattern from a large number of points on a graph

Let's consider a final note about using graphs to visualize possible relationships, to gain some insights or questions for further inquiry. When doing quantitative research, one will often have to "plot" on a graph the data for each person or each group studied. Computers can do this, and if there aren't more than a few dozen points to plot, a person may do this on their own. Let's go back to the hypothetical example of studying people's level of income in relation to their age. If the data have already been analyzed and you know that, "on average" 30-year-olds earn a certain amount, 31-year-olds earn another amount, then you can plot the appropriate income level for each age group on the graph and draw the line from age 30 to 31, and so forth to 65, if you're study ages 30 to 65, for example. However, if the data have not yet been summarized for you, and you have information for say, 100 individuals of various different ages and incomes, then in this case, you have to draw *a point* on the graph for each person. Each point represents the person's age in combination with their income—that is, a value on the x-axis and a value on the y-axis. The graph will look a lot like the scatterplot diagram below (see Figure 9.6).

Let's suppose, further, that the black dots represent a person's income in relation to their age, and the gray dots represent their height in relation to their age. Note that the gray dots are spread pretty much "all over the place" on the chart above; there is no clear pattern between age and height (people grow until their early 20s and pretty much don't shrink in height too much until they are more elderly). However, the black dots, while they are somewhat "all over the place" do still cluster along the straight line that has been drawn on the graph. This straight line is a sort of "estimate" of the relationship indicated by the many black points. Overall, it seems that perhaps (in our hypothetical example) that income increases with age,

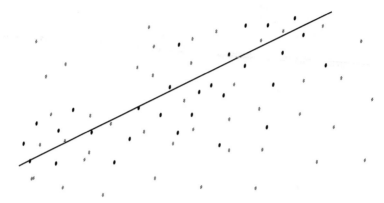

FIGURE 9.6 A scatterplot graph approximating a linear relationship.

and does so steadily (in a linear, straight line fashion), but the relationship is far from clear cut, and certainly there are many other variables that make a difference.

So, a strength of the use of statistics and numbers, especially if we use the visual aids of graphing, is that they sometimes do suggest some *possible patterns and relationships,* and we can follow up on these suggestions with qualitative research, further inquisitive action, and even additional quantitative research.

The uses, misuses, and abuses of statistics

Some of the advantages and uses of statistics

Statistics provide a *simplified way* of talking about complex qualities, by describing the qualities in quantitative terms, although as previously discussed, the validity of quantitative representations of complex variables (individual characteristics or social circumstances) is often tenuous and far from accurate. Examples are:

- the uses of IQ tests to measure intelligence;
- the use of age to estimate the extent of a person's experience, physical health, and/or social or developmental status;
- the use of blood pressure to estimate cardiovascular health;
- the use of psychological testing to characterize mental health, personality traits or inclinations; and
- the use of course grades to describe a student's learning and academic achievement.

Statistics can be useful to summarize information about groups in a *shorthand way,* or to *estimate* characteristics of a population—for example, a very large group of people, or a number of organizations of a certain type (e.g., schools or community health agencies), or a number of similar situations (e.g., what happens to people after a natural disaster or during an economic downturn), and doing so, without having to study the entire group. So, the researcher will study a smaller sample that they try to select to be representative of the diversity contained within the entire population. This saves time and helps one get to a main, manageable point. Examples of this are seen in opinion polls, in psychological studies that try to generalize about certain "types" of people by studying a small group of people who seem that they might be representative of the variety found in the general population.

In practice, getting a "good" sample is not easy, and previously, in Chapter 6, I discussed the importance of sampling for diversity. I learned from my long-time colleague Terry Lunsford that the famous historian of statistical methods, M.G. Kendall, summed up the role of statistics as strategies for making meaningful statements about the world by studying only a small portion of the world. Indeed, generalizations are always made on data that come from just part of the realities that we are trying to understand.

Further, statistics can provide standardized, and easily repeatable, procedures for detecting relationships between groups—for example, for comparing two groups of people in terms of their health or mental health, or for comparing two different treatment programs to see if one is more "effective" than another in accomplishing certain goals. This was illustrated above with the hypothetical example of a study of the impact of Public Service Announcements in educating people to limit their consumption of sugary beverages. Assuming we use such statistical procedures with an open mind, we may detect patterns in a complicated mass of information, which might otherwise go unnoticed or be "incorrectly" interpreted because of our biases. The mathematical methods provide us with some standards for evaluating the extent to which we should be confident in our perception of certain patterns in the data. So, considering another example, one could perhaps study the perception that certain family circumstances are a central factor in giving rise to a particular type of mental illness, by comparing the incidence of mental illness among people in different types of family conditions.

In my experience, statistical methods are especially valuable in helping us to think about possible patterns or relationships to investigate further. In particular, I believe that visual aids such as bar graphs, pie charts, and lines connecting data points on a graph can be especially helpful to further stimulate our thinking, and push our inquiry forward. Nevertheless, I'm reluctant to draw conclusions from quantitative data, unless I can also consider detailed, nuanced qualitative information as well.

The varied and qualitative meanings of any number

An important thing to keep in mind is that numbers are always associated with imprecise and qualitative meanings, and statistics can sometimes be illuminating, but also oftentimes overly simplify, or even misrepresent, whatever we are trying to understand.

I have been encouraging us to think about numbers as being similar to words and concepts. Just like words and concepts, the *meaning* of a number may change depending upon our purposes in using it, and the context in which we are using it. Like words and concepts, when we use numbers, we are usually doing so to think and communicate about their *relationship* with another word or concept. Although we can talk about the number "2" in the abstract, in everyday life we typically talk about "two of *something*"—two cans of soup, two times we observed the same thing, 2 years old (age), 2 feet long (distance, or height of a particular object). Further, when we use the number "two" there may still be questions or details left unanswered. Two cans of soup—but what kind of soup? How large are the cans? Two years old—but what are we talking about? Are we just sharing the age of our child or friend's or relative's child? Are we making a point about what we observe or perhaps expect by way of behavior from a child that's two years old? In actual everyday life, *using numbers to describe something should raise as many questions as it provides answers.*

So, my perspective is that numbers can be valuable and useful, *and* we should use them to raise more questions, to stimulate further critical reflection and curiosity, not to "end" our inquiry or study of something. In other words, *our quantitative descriptions and characterizations of things should push us to reach for deeper, qualitative understandings.*

Related to this, statistical methods and numerical measurements are no substitute for our own judgment. To do transformative action-and-inquiry, we must use our experience and previous observations, our open-mindedness and curiosity, our intuition and ability to make interesting speculations, our theoretical knowledge and understanding of the facts in our fields, and probably good old-fashioned common sense, too. We will need to continually ask ourselves such questions as: what do we want to measure and why? What is a "good" measure of this? What are the limitations or problems with measuring "this"? What different, and varied, real world interpretations of events might account for this particular statistical result? Or, for that matter, why was this particular statistical method appropriate, and perhaps also limited—keeping in mind our purposes and the nature of whatever it is we are studying?

Some limitations of statistics

They can oversimplify. For example, grades summarize the complexity of all that a person learns in a class into one symbol, even though they may have learned much in one area, and very little in another way. IQ tests can oversimplify because there are many different types of human intellect, and consequently, ways of exercising "intelligence" cannot be so neatly summarized in one concept or measure of "intelligence." Furthermore, it has been shown that there are many cultural biases and other problems of "validity" that call into question the accuracy, the meaningfulness, and usefulness of these "intelligence" tests.

Similarly, cost-benefit equations often risk reducing profound human events and conditions, such as health, learning, and even life and death, to dollars and cents. The tendency to do this kind of quantitative oversimplification can be traced in part to certain historical trends and forces, and the efforts by some to view "dollars and cents" as the main criterion of what is of "value" in our lives. However, it is not an obvious "fact" or "truth" that decision-making about what is valuable in life should be boiled down to units of economic currency.

Estimates about groups or individuals are not so useful in helping us to make predictions or judgments about individuals, or specific events, without additional information about the particular individual or circumstances with which we are concerned. For example, we have never met Joe but must greet him in an airport. We know that Joe plays on a basketball team and their average height is 6' 7". Do we look for someone quite tall, at the risk of overlooking a shorter person (who might play basketball) and who has that look on his face that he is looking for someone he has never met but who is supposed to be meeting him in the airport? Or, to take a different example, suppose that emotionally troubled people get certain scores on the MMPI (a personality test that assesses the likelihood of an emotional disturbance), similar to the scores of someone we know, perhaps as a client, named "Bob." Should we then assume that Bob is very disturbed, as well? How do we use this information, while still being curious to learn about other, relevant but perhaps contradictory information?

Mathematical methods are just aids to help us with the very complex, and multifaceted, process of drawing inferences and making judgments about how to make sense out of a lot of information. *Numbers can't make the decisions for us.* We must understand why, based on present information and past knowledge available to us, a particular method *might* be the "right" one to use. Further, we need to critically examine the "reasonableness" of whatever conclusions we draw from mathematical computations. If we knew nothing about freeway driving, what might we conclude from the statistical "finding" that a very large percentage of cars start blinking on the right side of their tail lights just as they reach a certain 100-yard stretch of the freeway?

To consider a different example, we could compare through statistical tests the exercise habits of hospitalized people with those not hospitalized in a particular year to test the importance of exercise for health. If hospitalized people exercise less, does that mean that lack of exercise was the main factor causing them to be in the hospital? Perhaps, to some extent. Maybe it's also quite likely that people who are ill enough to stay in the hospital might not be well enough to exercise? There are of course many other ways we could improve our thinking about how to "statistically test" the importance of exercise to health. People who do long-term studies "track" people of the same age group, and with other similar and various characteristics, for many years. Then, perhaps after years, they will see some patterns. Perhaps those who don't have to stay in the hospital do, on average, exercise more. But let's also look at the exceptions. What can we learn from the histories of those who exercise very little, but end up being healthy for many, many years? What about the histories of those who exercise a lot, but end up with some major illnesses? What can we learn from their stories? In this light, statistics provide a nice introduction for our inquiry, and not so much a "conclusion."

Quantitative and qualitative approaches to research can work together very well, in many cases—especially, if we are mindful of, and practice, some of the important qualities of transformative action research. That is the focus of the next section of this book.

Note

1 https://towardsdatascience.com/statistical-tests-when-to-use-which-704557554740; https://www.khanacademy.org/math/ap-statistics/tests-significance-ap/idea-significance-tests/v/p-values-and-significance-tests; https://hbr.org/2016/02/a-refresher-on-statistical-significance/

PART III
Important considerations in doing transformative action research

In Part III, I focus on several "qualities" of what I see to be "good" action research, qualities which may otherwise be overlooked or underrated, as is all too often the case in professional and scholarly research and writing. In Chapter 10 on "The immediate tasks and the bigger picture," I discuss the importance of not only focusing on the practical and immediate problems that are apparent and urgently before us today, but also of paying attention to the oftentimes invisible, but important "bigger picture" and "longer-term" issues before us. Today, some of us have come to realize that the large-scale problem of the climate emergency cannot be ignored by our attending only to immediate problems. I also suggest that accelerating inequality in our society, powered and supported by our neoliberal economic system, is another bigger picture dynamic that we cannot ignore. (To learn more, read the article, and look at the short video, "The Truth about Privatization", by Robert Reich, former US Secretary of Labor and Chancellor's Professor of Public Policy at the University of California at Berkeley and Senior Fellow at the Blum Center for Developing Economies: https://www.nationofchange.org/2018/12/13/the-truth-about-privatization/#.XBLcXORP-_k.email/.) To address these bigger picture issues while also paying attention to the many immediate daily challenges before us, requires a "both/and" perspective. Often, we might well decide to address short-term, immediate problems in combination with attention to larger-scale, longer-term problems. Furthermore, the immediate, small-scale and the longer-term, large-scale problems are often connected. Our action-inquiry must aim to study and address these together, as is also suggested in Chapter 11 on "Probing beneath the surface."

For example, today, as I finalize this book, the entire world is being swept by a coronavirus pandemic. Inquiry and action on this problem must be immediate, decisive, and well-informed. At the same time, we should not ignore further inquiry and action on understanding and transforming what this crisis is revealing to us, *if we look carefully at what has been there all along, but for many of us, out of view or "off our radar."* There is the climate emergency with the destruction of the natural habits of many species, among other factors, which many suggest have created conditions favorable for more mutating viruses and pandemics. The pandemic itself exposes raw what we should have already seen—the vulnerability of "have nots" to further deprivation—people who are overworked and underpaid, the homeless, the children living in poverty who rely on going to school to receive one solid meal per day, the crowded prisons in this era of mass incarceration, the underdeveloped public health care system which plays second fiddle to profit-making corporations in the health care industry. Transformative action research must attend to the immediate and somewhat apparent, and also to the oftentimes even more critical, less well-seen underlying dynamics and challenges embedded in the larger societal picture. Chapters 10 and 11 aim to remind us to inform each action research effort with this type of awareness and attentiveness.

In a related way, Chapter 12 on community knowledge-building underscores the importance of soliciting, and even trying to mobilize, participation of others in our action research endeavors, be they large or small. Transformative action research takes the view that each person is potentially an important creator of knowledge, and of needed, enlightened action. This viewpoint builds on insights from Chapter 8 on the great value of collaboration in action research. Furthermore, it is of critical importance in developing a strong, and vital, democratic society. So, in order to not just do any sort of action research, but to do participatory action research, it is necessary to think in terms of the role and power of people from many walks of life in contributing to "community knowledge building." Finally, since transformative action research necessarily attends to one's values, ethical considerations are part of an action research effort, and this will be discussed in Chapter 13. Ethical considerations are important in designing research efforts. Whether we are doing a formal action research project, or everyday action-and-inquiry, we should be very much aware of our social responsibilities and the values supported or challenged through the consequences of our action research and inquiry.

At WISR I have collaborated with others in previously writing about some important guiding principles to keep in mind as we do action research "the WISR way," that is, as we try to do "transformative action-and-inquiry." It is worth highlighting some of these key principles and qualities, as an introduction to this Part III of the book:

- Inquiring into both the immediate tasks and short-term challenges at hand, and also the "bigger picture." This "bigger picture" includes other theories, readings, and especially longer-term and larger-scale societal issues and implications. This means not focusing on "trees" to the exclusion of the "forest" and the "landscape beyond the forest."
- Probing beneath the surface of what is first apparent to us, and aiming to not only describe what we see, but also to try to understand underlying dynamics that are often not so easily noticed.

- Taking one's own experiences and insights seriously, as a basis for thinking, writing, conversations with others, and larger action, rather than relying only on the knowledge from books and the ideas embedded in existing policies and practices within organizations, and for this reason,
- Seeing each person, and each group and community of people, as valuable sources of knowledge-building.
- Being concerned with human values and social justice, not with so-called value-free research, or with research and efforts which only serve the status quo. For this reason, as well, we must attend to the ethical consequences of our action research endeavors.
- Looking beyond ourselves, as well—as in doing reviews of literature and interviews with others—rather than assuming we can't learn from others, even those whose thinking or purposes we believe to be flawed in important ways.
- Telling, eliciting, and listening to stories and paying attention to tangible examples–not just using abstractions—as was discussed in Part II.
- Understanding and practicing "action research," especially "transformative action-and-inquiry," as an *evolving, emerging process*, where the steps in the process (discussed in Part II) intertwine with one another, and where the steps must be designed, and continually improvised on, throughout the process. This is in contrast to more conventional, formulaic approaches to research methodology.
- Writing and rewriting in our own voice—to think out loud with oneself, to communicate and share with others, to stimulate collaboration and participation with others, and to refine ideas and strategies (writing is part of an ongoing creative process, rather than an end point or an opportunity to set knowledge "in stone") (Bilorusky, Lunsford, & Lawrence, 2008).

I hope, that, by the end of Part III, near the end of this book, and as a prelude to the companion book on "cases and stories" (Bilorusky, 2021), that I will have helped you to have reached a much more grounded, deeply understood set of meanings for the flowing, ongoing process that I call transformative action-and-inquiry.

10

IMMEDIATE TASKS AND BIGGER PICTURE

Introductory considerations

(Revised and updated from an earlier paper with Dr. Terry Lunsford.)
In most community and educational organizations, the pressure of immediate needs is strong and continuing. We learn to deal with a series of crises, often, with lulls between them to catch our breath, and we may even establish a certain half-conscious rhythm of doing so, as a patterned workstyle. Even if not, many of us can become satisfied, for a time, with the tasks of responding to immediate needs, ones which we think are pressing and important. Consequently, we become absorbed in this process to the exclusion of seeing other ways and other dimensions of our jobs, including possible innovative efforts and community improvements. It's a cliché, by now, to say that we need to give ourselves chances, and occasionally the requirement, to look at the longer-range view, the larger aims and commitments we have, alternatives to the ways we become used to following. This chapter addresses some of these issues, and some ways that an ongoing, transformative action research process can help us deal with them.

We get absorbed and set into immediate reactions to short-term crises, because some circumstances spell survival or extinction for our enterprise. Others are less immediate, but we may learn to treat them, too, as crises, having learned how to handle crises by having to do it so often. And what is a "crisis," or more broadly an immediate need, that demands attention, is partly a matter of definition—of our sense of priorities, of what is worth spending time on, of what really counts in getting our most important jobs done, and keeping ourselves able to do them. It's important to define reasonable breaks and rest from the press of meeting demands. We need to do this to avoid what people like to call "burnout," visible and invisible. Furthermore, we may get satisfied with our crisis-orientation because short-run, technical and concrete problems are in some ways more manageable than the larger, long-range, more diffuse ones. We are surer that a short-range problem is a problem, and what it means, and what to do about it. Probably, however, we should also be attending to bigger picture, longer-term problems as well.

An action-and-inquiry process within our group or organization can be used as a focus for raising larger, long-range questions. That kind of process, as we have been exploring it, involves periodic or ongoing discussions of what our organization or group is all about, where it is in its development, what we have together learned from our experiences, how well we are meeting the intended goals, and how adequate those goals are to addressing our deeper sense of purpose and values. There are a host of other questions that may come up when we start asking those just mentioned. The issue of what larger and long-range goals and values toward which we are working is one such possible question. *With a transformative approach to action-and-inquiry, our goals and values themselves become a subject of inquiry and re-examination.*

Consequently, our action research must involve more than just doing a periodic evaluation of how well we are meeting stated goals, although that is a good place to start. It's partly taking a look at the goals themselves and critiquing them by reference to our larger values and deeply felt commitments. In addition, the "bigger picture" notion also involves something more like taking a step back and getting a whole new broader view on what we and others are doing. It's like lifting our eyes to the horizon, checking our surroundings, seeing how we fit ecologically into the rest of the world, so to speak. Sometimes, that can highlight new things in the daily operations of our organization or group that nothing else shows us, and such new insights can be powerful motivations for working out new ways of doing things.

Often, we may shy away from such "philosophic" issues as "What does it all add up to?"—fearing that the results will be inconclusive, burdened with wandering conversations and ruminations that serve only to encourage speech-making, and perhaps bring up divisive issues that make working together harder. Those are real problems, and they must be dealt with. We can aim to have systematic considerations, of what larger issues are impinging on our work. Again, getting beyond narrower, more clearly and technically defined problems makes things a bit messier. But it doesn't have to be chaos. One way of keeping the discussion concrete, for example, is by a discussion leader's asking people to tell how their experiences and thought processes have shaped their current views. That often helps to keep the discussion close to specific experiences, including shared ones that several people may know about, instead of letting the dialogue fly off into the heights of political or academic rhetoric, where we may just repeat what we've heard from others. At the same time, it can be important to let people have time and permission to grope for ways to express themselves, because otherwise many half-formed, but creative and insightful ideas may be lost to the group. And this can be especially true when "bigger pictures" are being discussed.

Strains between "everyday life" and larger contexts

(Revised and updated from an earlier paper with Dr. Terry Lunsford.)

Whether we realize it or not, there are a lot of implicit strains or tensions, or ambiguities, in the ways that our everyday actions and relationships fit into our larger values, and the bigger pictures of state, national, international, and other kinds of "larger" scenes. For one thing, we may all be agreed on working in fairly standard ways to help improve our community's health care, let's say, but we may do so for very different motives and with concerns for different emphases and agendas. Some of us want to help specific people, whom we see hurting. Some may want to learn about how health care really works in a community, to change the system for the better. Some may just want to work with other likeable people in a "good cause," and to earn a salary to feed their family's faces. Some may want to build a model of better health care that other communities can copy and change things on a larger scale. Some may be unclear about exactly what they are most interested in. Some want to help this group more, and some that group, when resources are scarce. So, we are faced with many dilemmas—what our larger values are, how they are connected to our work on an everyday basis, what should be the priorities and what might best be considered luxuries, what is possible and where can our efforts can best be spent?

Questions like these are always there somewhere, to be asked if we decide to, and the answers are by no means clear in any specific group that is working for community or educational improvements. That's partly why formal organizations, like nonprofit corporations, schools, and public agencies, have formally stated goals and charts of organizational relationships and rules. Over time, people have decided to do this, so that all of those questions don't have to be debated every time someone wants to do something. Still, the complexities don't go away because the organization chart says they do; they just change their form, and become implicit, sometimes hidden, sometimes too much for the group to deal with. Since we must deal with those ambiguities, anyway, we can at least turn them to our advantage, some of the time. Ambiguity gives us openness, freedom, opportunity to change. Looking at the bigger pictures can be a way to bring that freedom into play, to see new possibilities where we were stuck in a rut, before. By agreeing to an informal shift of efforts from one of our stated goals to another—for example, let's say, spending less time on doing things *for* people, and more on helping them learn how to do things *for themselves*, in a self-sustaining way—we can sometimes change our whole relationship to some larger issues in the society, and refresh our feelings about the way we work, in the process.

One of the issues that comes up again and again in organizations trying to improve communities is whether our short-range efforts to meet local needs are just "band-aids" for gaping wounds. Are we doing much to help people when we just help them cope with their oncoming crises, but leave them with the same pattern of crises to be solved? Is some of our work obscuring the problems that underlie the crises, by helping somewhat just at the crisis point, and making crises seem manageable? Would some other expenditure of our energies and efforts be a better way of making things better for more people, over the long run? When we ask these questions in the abstract, they raise all kinds of worries and possible problems; we can always shake our own confidence by thinking of what we are not doing. But looking carefully and thoughtfully at our specific activities, and figuring out how they fit into bigger pictures, can help us to get beyond those scares, and give us some answers that we can live with, at least until we get better ones.

For example, we may want to ask whether our ways of helping people make them less or more able to help themselves, thereafter. We may want to ask whether we are changing anything about the social relationships between people, the "social structures," systemic injustices, and processes that shape their troubles and the solutions available. Or are we only helping at the edge, on the worst crises that those processes keep producing? We can ask, how can we get better facts about the results of our work, which would bear on those specific questions? How can we identify the things that could be changed, if we put our efforts into them (such as, official decisions that could be made differently), and distinguish these from realities that we aren't going to change (like the coming of old age and illness to all of us)? An inquiry process that focuses on such questions and follows up with action to get better facts and shift priorities deliberately can make a big difference in the way a community organization operates. *The dialectics in such processes, between questioning and getting facts, between studying issues and doing something about them, are important, and they can help us to bring about important transformations in our practices and in our circumstances.*

Here's another issue; we should avoid merely hiring research specialists who may take over the process and convert it to their own uses. But, if we get the right attitudes going, over a period of weeks, months, or even longer, we'll start to find that we have co-workers who can be our colleagues in doing participatory action research as we do our jobs. And that can double our pleasure, while getting good work done. Ideally, we can further increase the participatory quality by involving community people in our agency action research, or by involving parents and students in school-based action research.

Looking for needed changes in the larger society and at underlying systemic issues

I have suggested ways in which we should look not only at the immediate tasks and challenges we face in our groups, schools and community organizations, but also look toward our longer-term efforts. Furthermore, the short- and long-term well-being and accomplishments of our organizations are still only part of what we should attend to. It is also important to be concerned with the "bigger picture" of needed societal changes that impact on the various specific tasks and purposes with which any socially responsible group is concerned. As C. Wright Mills wrote in the *Sociological Imagination*, people's "personal troubles" are connected to larger societal ills and underlying systemic problems (Mills, 1961). So for example, agency staff who are providing for the unmet, immediate needs of homeless people would be advised to try to join with those who are advocating for affordable housing and working on changing the social conditions that give rise to homelessness. Teachers who are working tirelessly to promote learner-centered education and multicultural inclusiveness in their classrooms might well look for support and opportunities to work with like-minded teachers and others who wish to strive for larger-scale social changes. One example is the need for improvements on such social policies as "No Child Left Behind" with all of its undue and oftentimes punitive emphasis on standardized testing, or for addressing limitations in state curriculum frameworks which, for example, give inadequate attention to environmental justice content (Bilorusky, K., 2020).

Some social theorists talk about these different levels of attention as "micro" (focusing on helping individuals), "mezzo" (interventions at the group level), and "macro" (addressing the larger-scale, societal issues). All three are important, and certainly given the many demands faced by those working in the areas of social services, education, or community development and organizing, it is usually not possible for any one person or group to focus on all three levels, or even two levels.

However, *having an awareness of how improvements and progress at any one level may be impacted, oftentimes, negatively by the absence of needed changes at another level is critical. Further, those who work at the micro or mezzo levels oftentimes have special, invaluable and detailed knowledge of the needs of specific groups of people who not only have unmet needs, but who also are likely to be marginalized by deep rooted societal problems and injustices. Their knowledge can be helpful to those working for macro-level changes. Hence, networking and collaboration among people working for change at different levels can be extremely powerful. Further, for those working for micro-level and mezzo-level changes, without an awareness of the impact of these bigger picture issues, their best intended efforts could end up being only "band-aids"* as many have pointed out for decades now. Temporary or imperfect improvements are not unimportant in alleviating immediate misery and difficulties, but they are not long-term solutions. *With a transformative approach to action research, we try to be very aware of the limitations of making improvements at any single level, alone.* Further, if at all possible, a transformative approach requires that, even when working at the "micro" or "mezzo" levels, we mindfully strategize ways of apportioning some time and resources for working at the larger, "macro" level, oftentimes most feasibly by joining with those involved in working for bigger picture changes.

As a brief introduction to developing the mindfulness necessary with a transformative approach, *there are at least three key domains of systemic injustice and major societal problems in which all of us should try to educate ourselves—racism, the growing inequality created by "neoliberalism," and the environmental emergency.* Much has been written about all of these but figuring out how to take on these challenges is not so easy. Making specific recommendations is beyond the scope of this book. However, I want to say a bit about each one so that they will hopefully be very much "on your radar" if they aren't already. Further, *I want to suggest in the strongest possible terms that ideally, any action research project will include as at least part of its design, some attention in beginning to address one of these three serious ills, or something of comparable, fundamental importance*. At the very least, we should join with others in dialogue about ways we can collaborate to take on some of the pervasive and deeply rooted ills.

It is too glib to state simply that racism continues to persist in our society, because it is pervasive and creates massive injustices in all areas of life. It is seen in the growth of mass incarceration in the U.S. (e.g., read Michelle Alexander's book, *The New Jim Crow*). The Southern Poverty Law Center is an excellent force combating not only racism but all forms of discrimination (https://splc.org/). There are many excellent books on "critical theory" which provides a valuable perspective that might inform most any action research project. One source is the book, *How Racism Takes Place* by George Lipsitz. As stated in the book's overview, Lipsitz

> contends that racism persists because a network of practices skew opportunities and life chances along racial lines. That is, these practices assign people of different races to different spaces and therefore allow grossly unequal access to education, employment, transportation, and shelter ... Lipsitz examines the ways in which urban space and social experience are racialized and emphasizes that aggrieved communities do not passively acquiesce to racism. He recognizes the people and communities that have reimagined segregated spaces in expressive culture as places for congregation (Lipsitz, 2011). *How Racism Takes Place* not only exposes the degree to which this white spatial imagining structures our society but also celebrates the black artists and activists who struggle to create a just and decent society.

Beyond racism there are other important ways in which people are discriminated against, marginalized and humiliated, and these include the deeply rooted injustice and discrimination based on gender, sexual orientation, ableness, religion, and economic class, among others.

Today, increasing numbers of people, many of them younger people, have the awareness and sense of urgency to discuss "climate change" or "environmental problems" by instead talking about the "climate emergency" as an "existential threat" to our future. The impact of the runaway destruction of the environment requires long-term, "bigger picture" initiatives, and as many experts have pointed out, we are running out of time if we wish to be successful in that effort. As critical as these "bigger picture," longer-term change efforts are, there are also some immediate steps that can and should be pursued, both to build toward the larger-scale efforts and to alleviate the serious ways in which environmental problems currently weigh especially heavily on some groups of people, especially marginalized groups. The field of "environmental justice" is concerned with how some groups are already unjustly experiencing every day the weight of this environmental destruction. Near my home, people living in West Oakland, and many areas of Richmond, California, and other low-income communities, are exposed to air pollution and other environmental toxins at very high levels. The results are that people living there, especially children, are at a much higher risk of developing asthma and other diseases. The impact of the lead in the water in Flint, Michigan is now infamous; and less publicized, but quite noteworthy, are the impacts of fracking on the health of people living in nearby communities, which are seldom if ever affluent.

Finally, I would suggest that in pursuing action research projects on many various topics, we should be mindful of the ever-present impact of "neoliberalism," today's dominant political-economic system, and paradigm in theory and practice. Since the 1980s especially, neoliberalism has been embraced by most of the powerful leaders of our two major political parties, and as a result, increasingly key societal functions—from education to prisons, and more—are privatized, operated for profit and beyond the sphere of public oversite and decision-making. Further, major functions such as telecommunications and mass media are increasingly under the control of corporate monopolies, with little room for any alternatives. This is especially problematic given our increased reliance on the Internet and TV for information and education. Neoliberalism, as an economic and a political system, gives priority to supporting a "free marketplace" over the role of government. Many have pointed out how neoliberalism is also driving the increased levels of inequality in our society (Reich, 2018; Klein, 2014; Jeffries, 2017).

Some analysts believe that neoliberalism as a political force and ideology was a response by the power elite to the governmental policies "Great Society" of the 1960s, and to the persisting economic and political priorities of the New Deal. The consequences of this powerful countermovement are that multinational corporations have been able to function freely and make greater profits, free of the restrictions imposed by not only the U.S. but by other governments as well. Ronald Reagan in the U.S. and Margaret Thatcher in Great Britain were leaders that ushered in the era of neoliberalism. In addition, in the United States, most, but by no means all, mainstream Democratic Party officials have supported neoliberalism to a significant extent, including Presidents Clinton and Obama. The policies that they have advocated have been less severe, and less "austere," than more conservative policies, but they still lean strongly in the direction of protecting corporate interests with neoliberal policies.

Further, in the same vein, the U.S. Supreme Court decision, "Citizen's United," has provided enormous advantages to corporations and their ability to have an unrestricted free economic marketplace. Less and less do individuals have the power through democratic elections to have a say in what the "bigger picture" of society will look like. Admittedly, this is the critical perspective that I have arrived at, after observing decades of intensified marginalization of so many people in the U.S. and around the world. Others may of course disagree. In the spirit of the inquisitiveness of transformative action research, I remain open to learning of meaningful and useful alternative analyses. I would strongly suggest that everyone at least seriously consider the possible negative impacts of neoliberalism on our lives, and on the lives of so many less privileged people.

Indeed, neoliberalism is so pervasive and powerful that it can often co-opt or even undermine some of our best intentions. Recently, my friend, Dr. Joyce King,[1] suggested to me the useful distinction between "transformative multiculturalism" (or inclusiveness) and "neoliberal multiculturalism." Without going into an in-depth analysis here, let me present some of my insights that were evoked by Dr. King's articulation of this distinction. Neoliberal multiculturalism conveys the view that institutional practices are "color blind," and that "inclusiveness" means the opportunity to compete in what is assumed to be the level playing field of the meritocracy. It *allows individuals but not groups of marginalized people* to become an "included minority," if one can check off a non-mainstream box to describe oneself on a job application. In the latter case, "being a minority" becomes a commodity to be used for personal advancement, so that ironically where many decades ago, one "drop" of non-white blood relegated one to being racially oppressed, now one "drop" of non-white blood or some other criterion of "differentness" can single one out for a relatively rare opportunity. Still, in the midst of these "opportunities" for individuals (leaving aside the issue of whether or not some people might exaggerate the relevance of their "differentness"), the oppression and marginalization of many groups continues and even increases dramatically. This is especially the case for African Americans and Native Americans, but also true for some other groups as well.

Providing opportunities for numerous "different" individuals to "succeed" in the political and economic marketplace is not transformative multiculturalism, nor is this genuine inclusiveness. It is a way to take this urgent matter of social justice "off the table" and hide it out of view. By contrast, transformative approach looks beneath surface appearances, and it aims to create fundamental, systemic, and longer-term changes. We have not taken a transformative approach to multiculturalism and inclusiveness, so long as African Americans and Native Americans are more likely to be impoverished, incarcerated, unable to receive adequate health care, more likely to experience major health problems, and be unjustly burdened and oppressed in many ways. Indeed, there are other groups, as well, who in various ways are oppressed and marginalized, including immigrants, and people from many other ethnic groups, people with non-conforming gender identities, those with physical and neuropsychological differences, among others.

It is beyond the scope of this book to provide an education in "neoliberalism," but the above-mentioned references and discussion may help those interested in reading and learning more. It is all too easy to give insufficient attention to pervasive forces, even powerful ones, because we are so accustomed to their presence. Those of us aiming to engage in transformative action-and-inquiry owe it to ourselves, to those with whom we are working and to those whose lives we hope to improve, to think deeply and critically to better understand the impact of neoliberalism. I believe this is critical if we are to rescue our hopes for a stronger democracy from the grasp of neoliberalism. Again, if C. Wright Mills were alive today, I truly believe that he would say that our "personal troubles" are often very much the wreckage resulting from the wave of "neoliberalism."

Note

1 Dr. King holds the Benjamin E. Mays Endowed Chair for Urban Teaching, Learning and Leadership at Georgia State University (GSU), and is past President of the American Education Research Association.

11

INQUIRING MORE DEEPLY

One purpose of action research is to make observations and analyses of the obvious issues and patterns of behavior involved with day-to-day community work or teaching in schools or colleges. An equally important, often neglected, focus is to look beneath the surface for issues and themes that are perhaps not so obvious and apparent. As discussed in Chapter 10, it is all too easy to get wrapped up in our routine activities, or what we first perceive as the immediate challenges before us, and then fail to look more deeply and more ambitiously at what we might accomplish if we inquire more deeply.

Probing beneath the surface in our everyday lives in organizations and communities

(Revised and updated from an earlier paper with Dr. Terry Lunsford.)
Daily occurrences are often the result of a complex combination of conflicting societal influences and individual motivations. In community and school meetings, it is not uncommon for people to have stated and unstated agendas. People may sometimes be very unaware of their own motivations and agendas, and other times, they may consciously pursue "hidden agendas." Similarly, most organizations have overtly stated goals and operational methods, as well as unstated and inconspicuous purposes, procedures, and practices.

For example, a stated purpose of public, two-year community colleges is to provide equal opportunity and access to low-income and minority students. Yet, as early as over 50 years ago, some educational observers suggested that a latent function of community colleges is to "cool out" low-income students (Clark, 1988). That is, while the overt purpose or manifest function of community colleges is to aid equal opportunity and upward mobility for low-income students, their latent or hidden function is oftentimes to convince these students that they should be satisfied to enter lower earning and lower status professions rather than to strive for further educational and career advancement. In discussing this contradiction between the latent and manifest functions of community colleges, we might find disagreements and uncertainty about the extent to which this contradiction is intentional. That is, to what extent do some people intend and plan the latent function and work to keep this function deceptively hidden from the surface view of community college functioning? If some people are behind such a deception, who are they and what are the different motives and social/political interests behind their deception? Are there people who unintentionally and unknowingly support this latent function? If so, who are they and what are the personal motivations and social influences which lead them, unwittingly into supporting this hidden agenda within the functioning of community colleges?

These are the kinds of questions we can ask ourselves as we attempt to probe and look beneath the surface. These questions help us to inquire into the sometimes contradictory agendas underlying organizational functioning. These questions also point us to the complexity of individual motivations, of our own motivations and those of others. Very often, as individuals, we are motivated by contradictory personal concerns and influenced by opposing societal pressures. We may not always be aware of these competing and conflicting inclinations, but at times we may be all too painfully aware of such inner dilemmas and stresses, but reluctant to reveal or admit these doubts to others.

So, probing beneath the surface is a way not only of better understanding our organizations and the challenging situations in which we are working for change but also a way of improving self-knowledge, and of better appreciating, the inner conflicts experienced by our colleagues, neighbors, and/or co-workers, even when we disagree with them. With transformative action research, it is best to assume—unless there is clear evidence to the contrary—that organizational activities often lead in contradictory directions and that individuals are motivated and influenced by conflicting tendencies. It is best to assume that while ideas, statements and agency practices may be taken partly at "face value," we must also look beneath the surface for additional, and often conflicting, aspects of the total reality.

To say this another way, there are different layers of meaning to any event, situation, or action. For example, in considering the actions of an agency administrator, there may be many different layers of meaning underlying any particular action. There may be their concern with professional prestige, a desire to protect the agency from external threats, a desire to keep a good image with community people, a concern for minimizing staff conflict and for making things run smoothly, a motivation to maintain "control," a drive to live up to their own self-image (perhaps as a leader with a democratic style of operating), and a wish to simplify the difficulties involved in doing their agency duties, to mention just a few of the possibilities. None of these possibilities are mutually exclusive. Many of these different possibilities may coexist as different meanings within an action. Similarly, we may note different layers of meaning underlying a group action. A decision by agency staff, for example, may reflect a desire to cover up disagreements, a shared commitment to certain social ideals and beliefs, a commonly arrived-at perception of what the path of least resistance is, a logical outgrowth of decisions made in previous meetings, and a rather superficial "agreement" which conveniently allows all the individual staff persons to pursue their own interests without being bothered or constrained by others.

Major societal trends and patterns of activity can also reveal coexisting, conflicting meanings. For example, consider the growing, and now widely accepted emphasis on "holistic" or "natural" health methods. The holistic health movement can be seen in a variety of ways, and as an outgrowth of many different social pressures and trends, and with different kinds of consequences. The holistic health movement may be seen as: 1) causing and/or resulting from an increase in public awareness of issues of personal health (including diet, matters of lifestyle, etc.), 2) an integration of the concerns of humanistic psychology with concerns of health and medical practice (e.g., the ways in which our emotions and psychological well-being influence our overall health), 3) an outgrowth of alternative lifestyles beginning in the 60s and continuing and building momentum over time, 4) an emerging and increasingly acknowledged area of professional practice (with its own schools, methods of professional licensing and status), 5) a logical extension of the American spirit of individualism with its emphasis on the idea that each of us controls our own destiny, and 6) an economically inexpensive alternative to the rising cost of health care which will remove the economic burden that the conventional medical profession (and the health care industry in general) have placed on "the economy" (that is controlled by the power and wealth of a few), among others. Depending on which of these meanings, or which underlying societal dynamics, we emphasize, we may then see holistic health as mainly "liberating" or as "oppressive," or as a complicated and sometimes contradictory conglomeration of both. A "both/and" option is that we may see the holistic health movement as both liberating and oppressive, and then we may be better able to develop some strategies that strengthen its liberating aspects and consequences, while minimizing the more oppressive dynamics.

Of course, our perspective may depend not only on what we have observed and noticed but also on our values and social/political interests. Consequently, we can only hope to develop such strategies and analyses by making concerted efforts to look beneath the surface and to examine the varied layers of meaning, and think about these various meanings in light of our values, experiences and observations, and purposes. A useful exercise for each of us might be to take an issue of concern, then probe beneath our initial surface impressions to see if there are some not-so-obvious dynamics that might be at play—that could add to our analysis of the issue and how to study it and act upon it.

A related kind of analysis involves assessing the unexpected outcomes of activities and programs, that is, by looking for the indirect and unanticipated or less obvious "side-effects." Many of us are aware of negative side-effects in medical practice, where so many drugs help one problem but then create others. But side-effects can be positive as well. For example, an effort by an agency to do better community outreach may also result in a more clear and coherent sense of purpose among staff.

In the process of discussing outreach, basic questions about purposes and goals may arise, be shared, and thoughtfully considered by the group.

In probing beneath the surface, there are some pitfalls to be avoided. There is the danger that preoccupation with one layer of meaning may blind people to a fuller picture of reality. For example, politically aware staff in a community agency may be knowledgeable about the ways in which inequalities and power imbalances in the society exert important influences on many areas of community activity. In considering the example above about the possible "cooling out" function of community colleges, it may well be that racism and sexism are important ingredients that contribute to this unstated function. However, even if that's so, if we want to effectively critique and change community colleges, we must not become so preoccupied, for example, with the racist and sexist dynamics involved that we are unable to observe and analyze other dynamics and layers of meaning, as well. This would in no way negates the importance of racism or sexism, but we may usefully ask and consider how racism and sexism might fit in with other processes as well. For example, it may be that the "cooling out function" is also related to the fact that the economy is not geared toward full employment, and certainly not to employing most everyone at a "high" level of professional status, function, and salary. This possible reality is of course related to racism and sexism, but it is not solely a matter of these dynamics.

For purposes of political strategy and public argument, there are some advantages to focusing on particular layers of meaning. Consequently, in the political arena, we may often decide to focus on racism or some other particular and pervasive social injustice that should be a priority, and perhaps also that at least some people recognize as a priority, and will then join together with us on action in that arena. Still, for purposes of critical analysis and careful observation, we need to be sure that we don't block ourselves from noticing and reflecting on many aspects and facets of any particular situation or issue.

Let's consider as an example, the increased attention that has been given to the causes and consequences of trauma, especially and increasingly, in the past 30 years or so. "PTSD" (Post-Traumatic Stress Disorder) is now a term familiar to many. This important broadening and deepening of professional and public awareness has led to many becoming engaged in transformative action-and-inquiry on the matter of "trauma." Many people are more aware of the long-term psychological consequences of war and are more concerned about the impact of child abuse and neglect, domestic violence, rape and other forms of sexual assault, and natural disasters. In many ways, there has been public collaboration in this inquiry, and many are probing beneath the surface to learn more. People are willing to be part of a dialogue if it involves them directly. Our growing awareness of the many facets of trauma and its consequences is an excellent example of "community knowledge-building" that is the focus of the next chapter.

In my view, much of the dialogue and the related inquiry, has been highly valuable and continues to lead to important insights and further recommendations for improved laws, policies, and practices. At the same time, whenever any topic becomes popularized and a topic of widespread discussion, it's easy for the guiding concept (in this case the idea of "trauma") to be become less "sensitizing" over time. Here's what I mean. Previously, we were unable to notice "trauma"; it was *not* a concept we paid attention to, and as a result, we were not "sensitized" to look for instances of trauma, and therefore not inclined to see how many people were in need of special help and support. Further, we were not so inclined to work for societal changes that might address the causes of trauma. However, now that "trauma" has become popularized, I would argue that there is a tendency to see trauma "everywhere" and related to that, to lose sight of how some types of trauma might be much more severe and problematic than others. So, trauma is now perhaps less sensitizing.

Such preoccupations with, even extremely important and profoundly pervasive, problems and injustices can hamper our ability to critically analyze and creatively act to change these deeper social realities with which we are so strongly and justifiably concerned. When a strong, valid, and passionate commitment begins to become a "desensitizing preoccupation," it may create a degree of tunnel vision that limits our own options for inquiry and action. *There is a sort of double-edged sword, here. As we learn more, the concept of "trauma" may become increasingly useful as "sensitizing concept," and also it may in some ways it may become a "desensitizing" preoccupation. If we approach our inquiry and our actions toward trauma with both curiosity and critical reflection, to probe beneath the surface, there's a good chance that the concept of "trauma" can continue to evolve and become more sensitizing and useful.*

Probing beneath the surface, we can see how not all traumas are "equal." There are one-time traumas that should not be ignored, but from which the survivor can likely escape and receive support, and where they can become reassured and where steps can be taken to prevent or minimize the reoccurrence of the trauma-producing event. A child who is bullied on the playground is quite likely traumatized by that experience, but it may be feasible to take prevent steps. This is not as traumatizing over the long-term as growing up Black in a society where one is likely to be aware that at any unexpected moment one might be harassed, arrested or shot by a police officer (be they a rogue officer or part of a massive culture of institutional racism). Informing the concept of "trauma" by noting, and critically reflecting on, varied instances of "trauma" then begins to create a sensitizing concept of "trauma"—a concept that grows over time, with a richer and more informative variety of illustrations. Trauma that is one-time and trauma that is institutionalized and "structural." Trauma that is hidden from the view of others and where one feels all alone and continuing to be vulnerable, as compared with trauma that is public, and further in contrast to publicly viewed trauma where there is a system set up to provide support and to take steps to prevent such future incidents. Trauma that seems random and unpredictable (e.g., natural disasters) and trauma that is continual and ongoing. One of my doctoral students, Diane Heller wrote an outstanding paper on the differences between those acts of interpersonal trauma (e.g., rape) that are perpetrated by someone who is sadistic and is consciously and intentionally trying to do harm as compared with trauma perpetrated by someone who is in denial that they are doing anything wrong. It is not that one trauma is necessarily "worse" than another type of trauma, but rather that *such differences matter* (Heller, 2000). Diane Heller's clinical observations were that they dynamics and processes that might most likely lead to healing of those traumatized were different (not necessarily easier or harder), depending on the mindset of the traumatizing perpetrator.

Further, as we have become more aware of trauma, we have become sensitized to what have become known as "microaggressions." This is extremely valuable, for many reasons—microaggressions do have negative impacts, and especially so when they happen to same people repeatedly. As we become more aware of microaggressions, we can become more aware of the systemic and institutionalized conditions, policies and practices will support larger-scale trauma. Noting the varied forms that trauma can take, and the varied causes of trauma, is very important.

Consequently, even with, and I would argue, especially with, a valuable and well-known concept like "trauma" we must make concerted efforts, through transformative action-and-inquiry to make trauma into an increasingly more nuanced "sensitizing concept"—with more illustrations, a wider variety of illustrations, and continued critically reflections into why those specific variations matter!

So, for example, if we are trying to study the concept, "trauma," we should not settle only on a 20-word definition, "trauma is … etc." Neither should we merely define trauma as, "what is measured by one's score on the "Such-and-such" trauma index or scale. For example, as useful as the ACES (Adverse Early Childhood Experiences Scale) is to make rough estimations of people's previous traumas, at best, it is a rough, initial point of departure for future research (Kelly-Irving & Delpierre, 2019). Starting off with a tentative definition of 20 words, more or less, is an ok place to begin, as is a well-developed approximate, quantitative index, but the concept must be re-evaluated, further refined and fleshed out with a *variety of specific examples of different ways in which trauma can be manifest or shown*. As we learn more and more about the variety of forms that trauma can take, how it can happen, what it looks like with some people and yet differently with others, then, over time, we can improve upon our "sensitizing concept of trauma." We will be able to improve on our briefly stated definition *and* the understanding of the definition and *what it can mean* will be improved by having a richer, varied array of examples of trauma to reflect on.

In our efforts to inquire beneath the surface, with curiosity and a critically minded attitude, the role of community knowledge-building can be exceedingly valuable.

12

COMMUNITY KNOWLEDGE-BUILDING

WISR's approach to action research centers on the idea that all of us must come to see ourselves as builders of knowledge, individually and collectively. In 1983, when those of us at WISR finished our three-year U.S. Department of Education-funded demonstration project on "Extending the Teaching, Learning and Use of Action Research throughout the Larger Community," we titled our final report, "Knowledge-Building in Everyday Life" (Bilorusky, 1983). Over the years, in our work with students at WISR, we have encouraged them to draw on their own experiences, and on the experiences of others with whom they are in contact, in inquiring to develop ideas and strategies that can make a difference. Some people call this "participatory research" where "researchers" are the people who are involved in trying to make a difference in the communities in which they live and the organizations in which they work.

It isn't just that I believe in each of us as knowledge-builders for practical reasons and because of my values, I also realize that the quality, solidity and validity of our knowledge, and the actions flowing from that knowledge, will be better—if it grows out of the experiences of many people, who by virtue of their involvements, are in a position to "know." Those with the greatest potential to become experts, including the builders of theories, are not distanced from what they are studying, but deeply engaged in all of the complexity and messiness of the problems and matters which are the content of the ideas they develop.

In discussing "community knowledge-building" as a key aim of transformative action research, we must revisit the perspectives and methodological approaches discussed throughout this book. Community knowledge-building requires that we use these recommended methods, such as learning with and from others, and collaborating. The result is not only "better" knowledge but also knowledge that can matter to people, and potentially make the world a "better" place.

Stories, tangible details and "sensitizing concepts," especially in participatory research

I wish to revisit here, now in the context of community knowledge-building, how important it is for us to make a practice of telling stories and listening for stories from others. Here is a relevant story that I heard, but never read. The story was told by J. Herman Blake, who was for a couple of years a faculty member at WISR, while also Provost of Oakes College at the University of California, Santa Cruz. Herman was not only an extremely accomplished academician but also an accomplished community organizer. He told me that Myles Horton, founder of the Highlander Folk School (Ayers and Quinn, n.d.; Horton & Jacobs, 2003) once said that it is *extremely important to "listen eloquently."* For me that powerful statement, which I use in the "dedication" statements for this book and the companion book, sums up one of the key ingredients of a transformative approach to action research.

Stories matter, and important concepts are often embedded in stories, or illuminated by them. An apt and well-told story can bring to life an abstract concept to make it understandable and useful, and to remind us of other stories which then begin to flesh out the concept. As more stories are connected to the concept, the concept itself becomes transformed over time, enriched, so it is no longer a simple caricature but a more complex and pertinent approximate characterization of the world. This "approximate characterization" of the world does not precisely define anything, rather it suggests interesting questions and possible qualities of the "concept." As discussed in Chapter 3 and again in Chapter 7, this is what sociologist Herman Blumer meant in advocating that in the social sciences we should use "sensitizing concepts" that combine general abstractions with a range of tangible illustrations of the concept (Blumer, 1969).

A decade ago, some of us at WISR collaborated with the Bay Area Black United Fund, helping them to plan and evaluate three major conferences, three Summits on health disparities in African American communities. A main point of the conferences and the evaluations was to bring people together to articulate their knowledge. What do they know about possible causes of, and solutions for, health disparities? Professionals and grassroots people, alike, primarily from African American communities, came together to discuss, ask questions, and share insights about the problem of "health disparities." People had their stories to share, their experiences and facts about these disparities, hopes for what could be done, frustrations, and much more. All of this added to knowledge about "health disparities," and indeed, the very concept of "health disparities" began to take on a new life and was transformed into a deep, rich, and textured understanding of health disparities, and the needs and possibilities for action. What emerged from this pooling of the knowledge and experiences of the many who participated in the Summits was a multifaceted picture of health disparities, and also of the circumstances and dynamics causing and resulting from these disparities. In writing the document to summarize this knowledge, the first thought was to call it a "white paper." However, true to the transformative spirit of curiosity and collaboration, the leaders of this effort had the insight to call the initial written product, a

"Black Paper." Three of those Black Papers can be found online (Bay Area Black United Fund, 2003, 2005, 2007).

Beyond the content in the Black Papers, an indication that substantial and valuable knowledge was emerging out of the Summits was the sense that many participants had that this conference was different than so many other conferences they had attended. Participants had the feeling that they were connecting with each other through the ideas and experiences shared. Many said it felt like a "family reunion." WISR PhD student, Barbara Cheatham, who was involved with the evaluation of the conference, observed that it was not the kind of conference where one just goes home and then files the notebook from the conference. People wanted to do something more with what had been started with the dialogue on "health disparities." In another context of more restricted, and less collaborative, inquiry, "health disparities," like any concept, could be just another abstraction—suggesting some relevant information, pointing out some trends and tendencies, but still quite static and not leading to much in the way of further thought or *action*. In this case, the idea of "health disparities" became enriched with the specific experiences, stories, images, feelings, and shared insights and beliefs among a group of people. As various specific connections and meanings became intertwined with the central concept during that shared, public, and collective process, the notion of "health disparities" became more dynamic and transformative. This led to new questions, new hopes, heightened and sharpened awareness of frustrations and challenges, new strategies of action. Some of the emerging ideas were not yet fully formed or completely clear, but there was great progress, intellectually, and in terms of increased collaborative engagement, energy, and follow-up actions. One of the initiatives was to organize a network of grassroots individuals designated as "Critical Mass Health Conductors," who received training and support, to do every day outreach to individuals, families, and groups in their communities, aimed at health promotion (https://www.youtube.com/watch?v=LjM0Lgd-1lM). That these African American Health Summits were so successful is also a testimonial to the value and strengths of participatory research and community knowledge-building for action and change.

Good science, making it public and valid

There are many versions of science, just as there are many versions of religion. Throughout this book, I have explained how *some* mainstream versions of science hide behind pretensions of "objectivity" through practices aimed at adhering to standardized research protocols, such as precise and inflexibly asked interview questions, predetermined samples, and statistical computations to determine if relationships are meaningful. I have been trying to make the case that if we wish to use action research for valuable and transformative purposes, then we must use a variety of strategies—allowing for imaginative and intuitive improvisations in data-gathering, reflective analysis and interpretations of data, and seeking out new data in response to the emerging insights and questions. Rather than keeping the details of our methods obscure and hidden from public view, I favor our going to great lengths to share with others the ways in which we have arrived at our (always) tentative and imperfect conclusions, inviting input about new questions and directions for further knowledge-building.

In Chapter 7, I discussed a variation off of the famous story of the group of blind men who were trying to envision what an elephant looks like. The original version of the story has as its moral, that we are like blind men in that, as individuals, we cannot "see" the whole picture, or we only see it from a limited vantage point. I lamented that many conventional researchers adhere to the most mechanistic versions of science and try to solve the problems of "validity" and "reliability" by using formulaic procedures that often ignore the complexities of the reality being studied and upon which we hope to take transformative action.

Qualities of knowledge-building

From time to time here at WISR, faculty and students have considered how various people throughout history and in different cultures have come up with new ideas. We have noted the importance of looking at the development of ideas and knowledge in its social context. We have noted how sometimes these creative people have demonstrated special qualities:

- a desire to look at things that don't quite fit;
- an inclination to probe beneath the surface appearances of things;
- an openness to new thoughts;
- a spongy mind that is open to and in contact with others from whom they can learn;
- active curiosity; and
- a sense of wonderment about things that is not fearful of open-endedness.

For knowledge-builders, the questions themselves, and the act of asking questions, seem to free up energy from within, and give direction to their efforts at action-and-inquiry. As John Dewey noted, it may be more important to follow a sense of direction rather than to move toward a goal. Goals are fixed and external to us, whereas our direction, our path, emerges from us, allows for questions and may change as we continue to learn more.

In one seminar, we discussed how notions of creativity relate to our ideas of war and peace, and the flow of energy in our endeavors in life. One person suggested that war is our poorest attempt at the movement of energy, while peace is flow and movement of energy. Stagnation of energy may result from fear, trauma, unresolved anger, and grief. We noted that a good question for our ongoing reflection is, "what are the qualities of a 'better' question?"

We are adamant about people taking their own experiences and insights seriously. We encourage people to take notes about their experiences and insights, and then to write further about them. So, we don't have to only rely on knowledge of others. Still, we can look beyond ourselves to further refine, test out, and extend our own knowledge, by doing reviews of the literature and interviews with others, for instance.

As discussed in Chapter 8, it can be very useful to write to communicate with others, to learn with others, to think out loud and fine-tune our ideas with others, and all the while striving to find our own voice on topics that matter to us. Writing and rewriting in our voice is important—to communicate and share with others, to stimulate collaboration, to refine ideas and strategies, to formulate action with others. These various methods of transformative action research often come together, and do so productively and with great value, when we are engaged in community knowledge-building!

13

ETHICAL CONSIDERATIONS

This chapter is overview to some of the ethical considerations involved in doing any kind of research, including action research and participatory research. I certainly don't mean to provide any recipes for addressing ethical dilemmas and decision-making, but I do hope to suggest some ideas to inform, and guidelines that may be valuable food for thought. Most importantly, we should strive to be mindful and reflective of how ethical considerations may influence our action research, and how our decisions may result in consequences for better and/or for worse. It is not possible to be value-free. Ethical problems are indeed more likely to arise if we are unaware of the ways in which our values impact our action research. Ideally, the purposes of any action research effort are informed and guided by our values, although hopefully also, not limited by our values. A transformative approach also requires that we question, re-evaluate, and in some cases, reformulate either the specific purposes of our project, or even the larger values that led to our initially stated purposes.

This chapter also addresses some ethical problems that arise when certain, key values—acknowledged widely by most scholars, professionals and "ordinary" citizens—are not embraced and used in evaluating the details of our action research aims and activities. These values, and the strategies for assuring that we attend to them, are discussed in the first two sections, on "Ethical issues in protecting research participants" and "Ethical issues in formulating the purposes and design of an action research project." The last section of this chapter takes on bigger picture concerns of the "social responsibilities" of our pursuing transformative action research. That discussion is only a brief introduction to some of the value-issues that I believe ideally should inform any action research effort. It is not in any way comprehensive but is meant to stimulate further thought on this extremely important matter.

Ethical issues in protecting research participants

Some specific ethical concerns in doing research are reduced in those participatory research projects, when participants are collaboratively engaged in those projects, are also well-informed of any risks to them, and are likely to benefit from the action research. Still, any action research endeavor, even with a strong participatory component, has uncertain outcomes, risks, and benefits to the people involved. So, many ethical considerations remain. Discussed below are some essential safeguards that those doing action research must be responsible to maintain. Further, when the action research is pursued in the context of a school, community organization, or public agency, there are Federal mandates for having oversite provided by an Institutional Research Board (IRB). A discussion of the details involved in the creation and operation of an IRB are beyond the scope of this book, so the reader is advised to review some relevant sources.[1] These Federal requirements and standards are based on three important principles: 1) Respect for individuals—this means, for example, minimizing any harm to participants or others, especially those with whom one interacts or about whom private information is obtained, and quite important with regards to vulnerable groups such as children, people who are marginalized, and those who are at risk emotionally. 2) Beneficence—where the benefits of participating in research outweigh the risks to participants; and 3) Equity and Justice—where no single group or groups are likely to benefit at the expense of another group or groups.

Key areas of needed safeguards are, with regards to respect

1. Privacy and confidentiality.
2. This can be particularly challenging in small social groups where it can easily be determined who said what. In writing and communicating their research methods and results, care should be taken to assure the anonymity and confidentiality of participants, unless participants explicitly give the researcher(s) permission to disclose their identity. This means, as well, that in writing up case studies or detailed examples of participant comments, the researcher(s) may sometimes have to change a few details about the case write-up or the person's comments, to prevent others from identifying them.
3. Disclosure vs. deception.
4. Concerns over the ethical obligation to disclose what one is doing sometimes conflict with the fact that people's behavior may change if they know they are being studied. This has been particularly problematic when studying less powerful groups. Researchers must be completely transparent with participants about the purpose(s) of their study, and that there not be any undisclosed "manipulations" of research participants.
5. Informed consent.
6. Research participants should understand what will be expected of them if they are to participate in the research. They should read, and be assisted in understanding, an informed consent form that is free from jargon and obscure

technical language. They should be assured that their participation is completely voluntary with no negative repercussions should they decide not to continue. It is also important that they are explicitly informed that if, at any point in their participation (including for example, during an interview) they feel uncomfortable, or otherwise decide they wish to no longer participate, they always have the option of immediately ending their participation. In addition, for example, with survivors of trauma or others who may be psychologically vulnerable, participants should be informed that if they feel that their participation has raised difficult emotional issues for them, and feel they may then need psychological support or counseling assistance, then they should inform the researcher who will then give them one or more referrals for support and/or assistance.

Key considerations with regards to beneficence

1. Likely benefits to participants should outweigh the risks. Ethical research has a strong likelihood of having greater benefits to participants and fewer significant risks. Even when participants are well-informed and provide consent, there should be some likely, worthwhile benefits to the participants. Possible benefits include 1) becoming better informed, either through the interview process itself, and/or later receiving a copy of the main insights and/or results from the research; 2) having good reason to believe that the research will contribute to worthwhile societal changes or community or organizational improvements that are valued by the participants; and 3) becoming better connected with others in their community or organization as a result of the action research project, among others.

Justice and equity

This means, for example, that participants are chosen for their value to the potentially worthwhile, and openly stated, purposes of the action research project, not because they are vulnerable or can easily be manipulated into participating. One group of people should not be exploited or manipulated in a research study to provide insights that benefit other groups. In particular, people from marginalized groups should not be research participants for research that will provide the greatest benefits to more privileged groups.

Consequently, anyone who makes decisions about the aims, design or conduct of an action research project may find useful the following a *partial* checklist of circumstances, or steps, requiring special attention by researchers, in order to be attentive to the welfare of individuals participating in the project:

a. when vulnerable populations, such as young children, prisoners, or the cognitively impaired are involved;
b. if there is any possibility of physical harm to any individual;

c. when posing sensitive questions, including topics related to sexual activity; victimization, use of alcohol or illegal drugs, or involvement in illegal activity;
d. by ensuring anonymous data collection so that the data are not linked to individuals;
e. requiring that information identifying individuals be kept separately from the information collected from those individuals; and
f. requiring destruction of non-research data at the end of the course or within a short time afterward.

Ethical issues in formulating the purposes and design of an action research project

Beyond protecting those who participate in any research, if we are initiating an action research project, or any research project, for that matter, we should be very self-aware about our motivations that might be influencing their project's goals and the decisions about how to choose and construct our research methods. If we are not self-aware, there are at least three dynamics that have the potential to undermine our action research's ethical integrity, the validity of our findings, and the value of our actions:

- Influence by funding and by those to whom we may be ultimately accountable. When conducting research funded by an institution, foundation, or company, the goals of the funder may conflict with needs to protect subjects, or actual research findings—for instance, if the institution funding the research is implicated in creating the problem studied. Further, there are risks that the project might become poorly designed and implemented in order to learn and accomplish things that fulfill the funder's agendas.
- Our "bias" in data selection and interpretation.
  We must continue to ask ourselves, how do our assumptions and expectations shape what we pay attention to? Which data do we include or exclude? How do we interpret the data? To what extent do our own, unexamined needs or agendas inappropriately influence our stated purposes and values in designing and implementing the project?
- Fraud and self-serving motivations.
  Career and prestige motivations have led some to fraudulently report research findings or more subtly, to influence the ways in which the research is conducted, for example, as noted above, with data selection and interpretation.

"Social responsibility" and transformative action research

"Social Responsibility" is a tricky phrase—it can mean quite different things to different people, just as its cousin, the "public interest" may mean different things. In pursuing transformative action-and-inquiry, "social responsibility" is a valuable "guiding concept," but one that is best used to raise issues and suggests lines of inquiry and critical awareness, rather than providing a clearly defined direction for action and research. In the previous sections of this chapter, I discussed how those conducting research, including action research, must be aware of the ethics of how the research may impact on those directly participating in the research. Beyond this, it is crucial that *we are responsible for the potential impact on the society, as well as on specific individuals and subgroups within the society, of the written results of our research and actions taken that may grow out of, or might be in any way influenced by, the research.*

A good starting point for becoming aware of our social responsibilities for our action research is by returning to the two of the principles related to points discussed above. However, in that section the principles only applied to the impact on research *participants*. *Now, we must apply those principles to the potential impact on all segments of the society, communities or organizations who reasonably might be anticipated as being affected by the research.* These first two guiding principles are:

1. Benefits of the research results and actions should outweigh the costs. Research and action research, especially, should aim to have, overall, constructive human and/or societal benefit(s).
2. Equity and justice should be aided. Similar to the points above, the benefits should not be unjustly or unequally distributed, especially if providing more advantages to an already somewhat privileged group at the expense of a less privileged or even marginalized group. This is an important qualifying consideration regarding point #1 above and point #4 below. Decisions about costs and benefits should, if anything, favor those most in need, most marginalized, and/or least privileged. If we err in the opposite direction, then equity and justice are not well-served. *"Social responsibility" must consider both "costs" and "benefits," and do so by consciously and carefully considering "equity" and "justice," and especially, to promote advantages for those who are already less privileged.*

Furthermore, we must be aware that cost-benefit analyses are seldom "straight forward" because the measurements of competing costs and benefits are usually not comparable. Such analyses are usually like "comparing apples to oranges" as the saying goes. For example, if some research suggests that a change in health care would cost the country $20 billion, but that 2 million lives would be saved, there is no way to use a quantitative analysis in making a decision about what to do. Otherwise, one would be deciding on what financial value to place on human life. There have been corporations that have made such computations based on the "profit-loss" model of economics—such as the infamous example of Ford Motor Company in their production of the Pinto automobile. Ford decided that the costs of wrongful death lawsuits due to a poorly designed and potentially explosive gas tank would be less than the cost of redesigning and rebuilding the dangerous Pinto model automobile (Dowie, 1977).

All too often, when discussing costs and benefits, advocates will only discuss what they say is a prohibitive cost, or a valuable benefit, without discussing openly and carefully, "the other side" of the *qualitative* equation. *Regardless of whether or not we are fully transparent, and whether or not we are fully aware and intentional, we end up making value-based, cost-benefit analyses in deciding upon what action research questions to ask, what problems to address, and how to act on the findings and questions-raised by our inquiry.* This leads to three more guiding principles to keep in mind in pursuing socially responsible, transformative action research:

3. Use qualitative, value-based decision-making. Cost-benefit analyses are always qualitative in nature and require that we make value-informed decisions. Decisions are not merely the rational outcomes of an "objective" or quantitatively measured process; they invariably require that we decide on priorities and "trade-offs" between what is often a complicated array of likely (or not so likely) costs and benefits. In wrestling openly and intentionally with what values to give priority to, we give others the opportunity to fully examine our decision-making process. This leads to the next principle.
4. Have transparency. As I discussed earlier in the book, all research should be transparent, so that others will understand, appreciate, and be able to critically evaluate, how and why we came to our research conclusions. When it comes to being socially responsible and ethical, it is especially important that we openly convey to others, our analyses *and our decisions about competing values, different types of risks, and the potential costs and benefits.* This leads to a further principle to keep in mind.
5. Weigh the *likelihood* of risks, benefits, costs, and research errors. It is impossible for any action research project to arrive at a conclusion or a proposed action with absolute certainty. Some research findings are extremely strong, and we can often say that it is extremely likely that if we do such and such, then some good (or bad) result we happen. Sometimes, a result is likely to be accurate for one subgroup, but we may know less about what will happen with other subgroups.

For example, with respect to levels of "uncertainty"—a program for "underachieving" youth in schools may be found to work really well for one subgroup, perhaps those who have a lot of parental support, but not so clearly work well for those with less parent support or for those who are frequently moved from one foster home to another. This doesn't negate the value of this as "general recommendation" or "follow-up action" but it does suggest that, based on the principle of "justice and equity," the implementation of this program should move forward only if it is also coupled with further investigation to learn what kind of program to develop for those groups who are very much in need, and for whom the results are not so clearly indicated to be "effective." Or, alternatively, we might look to see if there is a somewhat different program innovation that we can implement that is very likely effective with virtually all youth, even though the degree of effectiveness is somewhat less significant for the more privileged students who have considerable parental support. Based on the principle of "justice and equity," we might well opt to implement this program, while we continue to do research to identify two programs—one for those with parental support and one for those with less support—that are more effective for each of the groups. Once we accomplish that, if we are able to do so, then we would implement the two innovative programs, each targeted to the group with which it could be most effective and valuable.

Three other principles, also referred to in the previous section, are important in trying to be socially responsible in doing action research:

6. Avoid influence by sources of funding and authorities with power over us. Earlier in the book, I mentioned a consulting contract that we at WISR had with the redevelopment agency of a major city. They had obtained millions of dollars to build low-income housing aimed at serving the needs of low-income elders. Our instructions when beginning the comprehensive assessment of elder needs were to look at everything *except* housing, because that had been "taken care of." Subsequently, nevertheless, we pursued the kind of open-ended, widely exploring inquiry that we always try to do, and we ended up learning from many elders and service providers that housing was the single, most important unmet need. We investigated this further, and our data strongly confirmed this. This was highlighted in our draft report. The agency funding our consulting contract said that they wouldn't pay us for our work unless we took this major finding out of our report. I refused to do so, and this stalemate went on for six months before they finally accepted the report the way we wrote and paid us what was owed. A year later, I got a phone call from new staff at the agency—there had been almost a complete turnover of staff. It seemed that "somehow" a copy of our report was never kept in their files by the previous staff.
7. Address "Bias" in asking questions and gathering data. The example in point #6 above illustrates the importance of trying to be aggressively inquisitive in looking for all types of information and asking questions "out of the box." Our own assumptions, and outside pressures, can result in failing to conduct a wide, exploratory search for potentially relevant data, or to a narrow-minded or short-sighted interpretation of data.
8. Self-serving motivations. It is difficult to attend to matters of social responsibility, if we are overly preoccupied with how the research, or action research, will contribute to our career, reputation, or status. Even with sincere intentions, it is good to be aware of these sometimes subtle, but still significant, influences. Collaborating with others who have such awareness and sincere intentions is one good way we can work together to help keep one another "honest."

Note

1 https://www.youtube.com/watch?v=_UK5QatUEKE; https://www.youtube.com/watch?v=M6AKIIhoFn4&feature=youtu.b; https://www.slideserve.com/shanon/irb-submission-powerpoint-ppt-presentation

14

CONCLUDING REMARKS

Transformative action research is not a "thing"; it is more appropriately seen as a "sensitizing concept," as an organic, evolving process. In this book, I have suggested that "it" is characterized by a *coherent constellation of some key qualities, principles, and methodological approaches*. Also, it is necessarily a "work in progress" that should, and will, come to mean different things to different people. It is not "my" method or approach, but rather a set of related ideas, methods, and principles that I have learned from the insights of others, as well as through my over 50 years' of experience collaborating and being engaged with others, living and doing transformative action-and-inquiry. These concluding remarks are mostly reminders of points and notions that I hope you will at least reflect on and consider seriously. I fully expect that each reader will get something different from what they have read and considered here. Undoubtedly, for each of you some of these points will make more sense or seem possibly to be of greater value.

So, here are some potentially meaningful reminders for you to consider and perhaps put into practice, modifying each idea or method in light of your own circumstances, insights, and experiences.

- This book has been about "research," "inquiry," and "action"—and is an effort to portray an overall perspective for bringing us together in transformative ways to make a difference in our lives and the world.
- The word "transformative" is to emphasize how action research and inquiry can be used to bring about fundamentally new insights, practices, and change. "Transformative inquiry" as a way of living, involves bringing together thinking and acting in one's life, to bring about personal and/or societal transformations.
- Action research, or action-and-inquiry, is fundamentally about learning, and my decades of experience have convinced me that, overall, learner-centered

approaches to learning are most effective, especially because learners make use of what they have learned in ways that are significant and meaningful to them.
- Consider reflecting on what has been said in this book about:
    1. some of the key qualities of, and issues pertaining to, science and inquiry;
    2. how to participate and collaborate with others in inquiry;
    3. how to use and critically evaluate specific techniques and practices of action research; and
    4. ways to incorporate action research and transformative inquiry into your everyday life, and how you may help others to do this as well.
- Participatory research, and democratic community knowledge-building will be served if we try to develop among us a continually increasing number of professional and community participants who are knowledgeable about action research, and quite importantly, who can then help to teach others about transformative action-and-inquiry.
- The following strategies or considerations may often contribute positively to transformative action research:
    1. Being actively involved in the social realities, or circumstances, that we are studying.
    2. Considering alternative interpretations or hypotheses.
    3. Modifying and redirecting our research methods as we learn more.
    4. Using specific examples and stories to illustrate our concepts.
    5. Writing about our findings by "telling the story" of what we did during the research process, and how we came to our findings. In this way, we can try to be transparent about our methods, and potential biases, because when others read the story of our inquiry, they can decide whether, and in what ways, to take our research seriously.
    6. "Script-improvisation" is a valuable, guiding metaphor for transformative action-and-inquiry. All theories should be used as "scripts for improvisation," as potential starting points for further inquiry-and-action.
    7. Consciously and persistently trying to look for, find, and learn about examples that illustrate the exceptions to the rule, the variations on the theme. By understanding such "exceptions to the rule," we can better appreciate the "general theme" or "general rule," Through this process, we can then begin to develop a more comprehensive theory which accounts for both the examples that "prove" the rule, as well as those that are the exceptions.
- To take a transformative approach, it helps if we nurture these qualities:
    1. a desire to look at things that don't quite fit;
    2. an inclination to probe beneath the surface appearances of things;
    3. an openness to new thoughts;
    4. a spongy mind that is open to and in contact with others from whom we can learn;

5. active curiosity; and
  6. a sense of wonderment about things that is not fearful of open-endedness.

- Some valuable qualities that may contribute to the validity of our action research are:
  1. considering different situations and contexts, and the bigger picture;
  2. looking for specific examples to test out our insights;
  3. taking our own experiences and insights seriously, while also evaluating information from differing perspectives;
  4. looking beyond ourselves for information and insights from others; and especially,
  5. collaborating with others and getting the benefit of their analyses.

- Trying to adopt and practice these qualities, including transparency, is more important than whether we use numbers and statistics, more important than whether we adopt a particular research design, or any single research procedure. If we are transparent, then others will be able to evaluate our research, or action research, and decide how confident that they wish to be in our findings. Also, they can decide in what ways our findings seem to be "valid" and in what ways, limited.
- Sometimes emotions, as well as our idiosyncratic experiences, may actually aid the development of knowledge and expertise and be invaluable qualities of human intelligence.
- Transformative action research requires that we continually ask ourselves questions about what we think "matters" the most—about what's valuable, and what's useful or practical, in ways that matter to us.
- Science is a special version of abilities and understandings that we all have as human beings. It is a precious possession of all humans who want to participate in it. It can be reclaimed, at least in part, from the big research labs and academic departments that now dominate it. Seeing it as a social process, and as an important part of society, can be a step in that direction. Collaborating with each other in reclaiming science—that is, acting socially in another sense—is very much worth our efforts.
- In so many ways, our society and our culture, and especially those groups and people with the greatest power, influence and privilege, may significantly influence, and distort, our inquiry in ways that we may not always readily appreciate. Action research cannot realize its transformative potential without a consistent and continual awareness of the challenges involved in addressing these biases. For these biases are not merely "academic" matters that influence our "research conclusions," they impact our lives and our society, and especially the lives of those who continue to be most marginalized and least privileged people in the society.
- With the transformative approach discussed in this book, the following steps in the process of research need not always follow the usual conventional

sequence, but may continue to interact and interweave with one another throughout the process of action-and-inquiry:

1. asking questions;
2. sampling (where to seek data and information) and the actual data-gathering;
3. analyzing data; and
4. communicating what has been learned during the research, as well as of course, with action research, the important, additional step of taking action;
5. action may happen before, during and/or after the research, and ideally, we should remain conscious, of all three options for this sequence.

- We all observe, take in information, store it in memory, sort it into tentative categories, re-do these categories from time to time, come to conclusions, change our minds, re-interpret the ideas and facts we are using—and go on about our business as we are doing these things. Thinking together about these activities—what is generally natural about them, and what is special to "science" is important if we are to engage in transformative action-and-inquiry.
- As researchers, we are continually making decisions about what to look for next, what to sample for, or who to sample for, as the inquiry progresses, as we get more information, and as we do preliminary analyses of the data. The more we learn about our topic of inquiry, the more we know how to sample, to test out, and improve upon our initial ideas. It is important, to the extent possible to do "diversified sampling." That is, our understanding and ideas, and our actions, will be more informed and more "valid" if we try to get information from the range of people involved in what we're studying, or from the range of organizations or circumstances relevant to our research questions or purposes.
- In using statistics, we should not fall into the trap of abdicating our responsibility for, and opportunity to, weigh the evidence from many angles and then making the best judgment that we can, for now. We cannot rely on quantitative analyses alone. Very often there is an attempt to put effectiveness, risk, and effort into dollars-and-cents terms, so we can have a neat, and seemingly definitive, cost-benefit equation. But this is an artificial procedure. Instead, whenever we are in a position to decide, we need to take responsibility for making decisions, using our values and commitments, along with our best judgments in weighing what is often a very complex array of sometimes confusing, contradictory, or at least far from clear cut, evidence. Also, rather than translating qualitative issues into dollars and cents, we can begin to translate dollars and cents into human terms, and then weigh the evidence; that is, make judgments about the information available based on human and social considerations.
- We—those of us doing the research, engaged in inquiry—inevitably make judgments and decisions about data-gathering and analysis, whether we are doing so qualitatively, quantitatively, or both. In all cases, the solidity and limitations of our process should be transparent and subject to critical examination and evaluation by others!

- In using a "both/and" perspective, our efforts in "making sense out of experiences" becomes all the more interesting, less frustrating, and more important and meaningful. This doesn't mean that both perspectives have equal weight or validity, but that often, each perspective can contribute some things of value to our transformative approach to action-and-inquiry.
- It helps to have our perspective or "paradigm"—our value assumptions and considerations—consciously in mind, because we, and often others, will live with the consequences of our choices, for better and for worse. We do have a lot of freedom to pick our tentative conclusions, and our facts and arguments, to fit the values and purposes we want to serve. It should be added that if we wish our action-and-inquiry to be truly transformative, then we also have the challenge of intermittently re-evaluating our values and purposes, and our overall "paradigm" by seeking out "new" information and by considering fresh and new ways of looking at the data.
- It is always a good idea to get additional evidence, be it more quantitative or more qualitative, or both. The primary consideration isn't whether the evidence is "hard" or "soft"—because arguably all evidence is soft, and perhaps becomes a bit "less soft" if we are deeply and critically reflective in weighing the evidence, and also curious and imaginative in continuing to look for new evidence.
- Three related, important considerations in collaboration are: how to best communicate what we know to others, how and why we should collaborate with others to improve our research, and our action, and the importance of providing transparency about how we have arrived at our findings. Consequently, it is important for us to put ourselves at the heart of the story of the action-inquiry about which we are writing. This means sharing with our readers (or listeners) the thinking behind the decisions we make at various steps along the way when doing the action research, being transparent and engaging others in our thought processes during the inquiry. This includes writing to convey not just generalizations and abstract concepts alone but also to connect ideas and conclusions with a variety of specific examples. This means using storytelling, case studies and detailed illustrations—and, writing in our own voice and from our own perspective.
- With a transformative approach to action-and-inquiry, our goals and values, themselves, should become subjects of inquiry and re-examination. So, when a strong, valid, and passionate commitment creates a sort of tunnel vision, then it becomes a "preoccupation." In such cases, we limit our own options for inquiry-and-action.
- Even within our strong commitments, our informed critiques and analyses of social reality, and our primary areas of activity, we must continually look beneath the surface, to discern the many layers of meaning underlying our activities and the realities with which we are concerned. If we do this, we can become more effective and informed in our actions and in the pursuit of our commitments and concerns.
- We are responsible for the potential impact on the society—as well as on specific individuals and subgroups within the society—of the written results of

our research and of actions taken by others that may grow out of, or might be in any way influenced by, the research.
- We end up making value-based, cost-benefit analyses in deciding upon what action research questions to ask, what problems to address, and how to act on the findings and questions-raised by our inquiry. This is so, whether or not we are fully aware and intentional about it.
- When it comes to being socially responsible and ethical, it is especially important that we openly convey to others, our analyses and decisions about competing values, different types of risks, and the potential costs and benefits.
- Community knowledge-building requires that we learn with and from others and collaborate actively. It also importantly involves groups of people and communities coming together as builders of knowledge. Collective action-and-inquiry is important in a democracy, and in pursuing justice and equality. The result is not only "better" knowledge but also knowledge that can matter to people, and potentially make the world a "better" place.
- I realize that the quality, solidity and validity of our knowledge, and the effectiveness of the actions flowing from that knowledge, will be better if they grow out of the experiences of many people, who by virtue of their involvements, are in a position to "know." This means that as Myles Horton reportedly once said, "we must listen eloquently"!

Throughout all these endeavors we can try to adopt certain attitudes and frames of mind that aid this type of creative knowledge-building. So, highlighting here some of the previous themes; we should aim to:

- *Be exploratory, rather than narrow or habitual.*
- *Be reflective, rather than rote or unthinking.*
- *Be engaged, rather than aloof.*
- *Be inquisitive, rather than disinterested or accepting.*
- *Be collaborative, rather than disconnected from dialogue and participation with others.*
- *See ideas as emergent, rather than static and conclusive.*
- *See methods as necessarily improvisational, rather than formulaic or mechanistic.*
- *Have a sense of the "bigger picture," seeing not just the trees but the forest as well, and the landscape beyond the forest.*
- *Tell and listen to stories and tangible examples, rather than settling on abstractions, alone.*
- *Be concerned with human values and social justice, rather than accepting the myth of value-free research, which very often means research that serves, even if only indirectly, the status quo.*

More for the interested reader—brief highlights of what will be addressed in Volume 2—Action research: Uses and illustrations of transformative inquiry

As a follow-up to this book, the reader may wish to look at the companion book, *Cases and Stories of Transformative Action Research* (Bilorusky, 2021). The first part of the book describes and discusses the details involved in specific applications of methods and principles of transformative action research—1) program evaluations; 2) community needs assessments; 3) creating community-based think tanks; 4) engaging in day-to-day activities to improve organizations from within while also being aware of the importance of working for change outside one's organization as well; and 5) developing pilot projects and concept papers. There is also a discussion of the application of transformative action research ideas and methods to critically reflect on unfolding research and decision-making challenges and dilemmas, in the midst of the traumatic, rapidly unfolding uncertainties of the Covid-19 pandemic.

The chapters in the second section provide tangible and detailed illustrations of the wide variety of ways in which transformative action research can be used, including 1) as intellectual activism, for example in addressing the problem of workplace bullying; 2) the preservation and restoration of the traditional culture of the Omaha tribe, and successful current efforts to support and further the tribe's rights and the education of tribal youth—ranging from impacting a U.S. Supreme Court decision to increasing interest in and knowledge of tribal culture among Omaha children, youth and adults; 3) the use of participatory research in promoting cross-cultural collaboration among U.S. school teachers with indigenous educators, youth and other adults in Mexico and Central America; 4) one WISR doctoral alum's story of how action research helped her to "get out of the book and into the world"; 5) the similarity of this approach to transformative action-and-inquiry with the efforts of innovative college professors to teach physics as inquiry; 6) discussion of a project under way aimed to explore how "Artificial Intelligence-student collaboration" might well provide students, especially from marginalized circumstances, opportunities to develop higher order inquiring abilities, as well as valuable, practical technological skills and know-how—while also expanding our understanding of the uses and limitations of AI; 7) vignettes describing and commenting on a variety of action research projects successfully pursued by WISR learners over the years, along with their comments on their experiences; and 8) finally, an autobiographical analysis of how my experience and understanding of inquiry-and-action has evolved from childhood to old age, and the role of other people and social circumstances in promoting my own learning of transformative action research. With these reflections, I try to illustrate some of the many ways in which "social learning" from and with others can be key to expanding one's abilities and understanding of inquiry, if one is fortunate enough to find their way into situations ripe with opportunity.

REFERENCES

Alexander, M. (2012). *The New Jim Crow*. New York: New Press.
Ayers, B., & Quinn, T. (n.d.). Myles Horton (1905–1990). Retrieved May 21, 2020, from https://education.stateuniversity.com/pages/2072/Horton-Myles-1905-1990.html
Barrett, J. (2020, March 30). Stanford professor: Data indicates we're severely overreacting to coronavirus. Retrieved May 20, 2020, from https://www.stress.org/stanford-professor-data-indicates-were-severely-overreacting-to-coronavirus
Bay Area Black United Fund. (2003). Bay Area African American Health Initiative – 2003. Retrieved May 20, 2020, from https://issuu.com/baaahiblackpapers/docs/blackpaper_2003
Bay Area Black United Fund. (2005). Bay Area African American Health Initiative – 2005. Retrieved May 20, 2020, from https://issuu.com/baaahiblackpapers/docs/blackpaper_2005
Bay Area Black United Fund. (2007). Bay Area African American Health Initiative – 2007. (2007). Retrieved June 20, 2020, from https://issuu.com/baaahiblackpapers/docs/black_paper_2007.pdf
Becker, H. S. (1958). Problems of inference and proof in participant observation. *American Sociological Review*, 23(6), 652–660. doi:1958-ProblemsOfInferenceAndProof.pdf
Becker, H. S. (1963). *Boys in white: Student culture in medical school Howard S. Becker*. Chicago: University of Chicago Press.
Becker, H. S. (2017). Problems of inference and proof in participant observations. *Sociological Methods*, 398–412. doi:10.4324/9781315129945-35
Becker, H. S. (2018). *Outsiders: studies in the sociology of deviance*. New York: Free Press.
Becker, H. S., Geer, B., & Hughes, E. C. (1995). *Making the grade: The academic side of college life*. Piscataway, NJ: Transaction.
Benner, P. (2001). *From novice to expert: Excellence and power in clinical nursing practice*. Upper Saddle River, NJ: Prentice Hall.
Bilorusky, J. A. (1972). Reconstitution at Berkeley: The quest for collective self-determination. Unpublished Doctoral Dissertation. University of California, Berkeley.
Bilorusky, J. A. (1975). *Improvisational competency-based learning: Exemplars from personal experience*. Lecture presented at 30th National Conference of the American Association of Higher Education, Chicago.

Bilorusky, J. A. (1983). *Knowledge-building in everyday life: Final report to the U.S. Department of Education, Fund for the Improvement of Post-secondary Education. Nationwide demonstration project – "Extending the teaching, learning and use of action research throughout the larger community. 1980–1983"*. Berkeley, CA: Western Institute for Social Research.

Bilorusky, J. A. (2020). Mobilizing & coming together during the coronavirus. Retrieved May 20, 2020, from https://www.wisr.edu/mobilizing-coming-together-during-the-coronavirus/

Bilorusky, J. A. (2021). *Cases and stories of transformative action research: Five decades of collaborative action and learning.* Routledge.

Bilorusky, J. A., & Butler, H. (1975). Beyond contract curricula to improvisational learning. In N. R. Berte (Ed.), *Individualizing education through contact learning*. Tuscaloosa, AL: University of Alabama Press.

Bilorusky, J. A., & Lawrence, C. (2003). Multicultural, community-based knowledge-building: Lessons from a tiny institution where students and faculty sometimes find magic in the challenge and support of collaborative inquiry. In T. D. Dickinson (Ed.), *Community and the world: Participating in social change* (pp. 63–81). New York: Nova Science.

Bilorusky, J. A., Lawrence, C., & Lunsford, T. (2008). Participatory action research, inclusiveness, and empowering community action at the Western Institute for Social Research. In T. D. Dickinson, T. A. Becerra, & S. B. Lewis (Eds.), *Democracy works: Joining theory and action to foster global change* (pp. 19–38). Boulder, CO: Paradigm.

Bilorusky, K. (2020). Evaluating environmental justice in K-12 schools. Senior Honors Thesis. College of Natural Resources, University of California, Berkeley.

Bilorusky, N. (2020). Multicomponent interventions to reduce future incarceration for children with early-onset conduct disorder. Senior Honors Thesis. Department of Social Welfare, University of California, Berkeley.

Blumer, H. (1969). *Symbolic interactionism: Perspective and method.* Englewood Cliffs, NJ: Prentice Hall.

Blumer, H. (n.d.). What is wrong with social theory? Retrieved May 17, 2020, from https://www.brocku.ca/MeadProject/Blumer/Blumer_1954.html

Butler, H., & Bilorusky, J. (1975). Experimenting community: A new curriculum for human service professionals. *Education and Urban Society*, 7(2), 117–139. doi:10.1177/001312457500700202

Butler, H., Davis, I., & Kukkonen, R. (1979). The logic of case comparison. *Social Work Research and Abstracts*, 15(3), 3–11. doi:10.1093/swra/15.3.3

Cavalier, D. (2011). Scientists tap the wisdom of crowds. *Discover Magazine*, (January/February), 74.

Clark, B. R. (1988). *Educating the expert society.* San Francisco, CA: Chandler Publishing.

Dewey, J. (1968). *Democracy and education: An introduction to the philosophy of education.* New York: Free Press.

Dewey, J. (2015). *Experience and education.* New York: Free Press.

DiStefano, A., & Rudestam, K. E. (2007). *Encyclopedia of distributed learning.* Thousand Oaks, CA: Sage.

Dowie, M. (1977). Pinto madness. Retrieved May 20, 2020, from https://www.motherjones.com/politics/1977/09/pinto-madness/

Dreyfus, H., & Dreyfus, S. (1985). From Socrates to expert systems: The limits of calculative rationality. Retrieved May 17, 2020, from www.psych.utoronto.ca/users/reingold/courses/ai/cache/Socrates.html

Dreyfus L., & Wrathall, M. A. (2016). *Skillful coping: Essays on the phenomenology of everyday perception and action.* Oxford: Oxford University Press.

Dreyfus, S., & Dreyfus, H. (1979). The scope, limits and training implications of three models of aircraft pilot emergency response behavior. Retrieved May 17, 2020, from https://www.

researchgate.net/publication/235032293_The_Scope_Limits_and_Training_Implications_of_Three_Models_of_Aircraft_Pilot_Emergency_Response_Behavior

Fanon, F. (1967). *Black skin, white masks*. New York: Grove Press.

Freire, P. (1972). *Pedagogy of the oppressed*. New York: Herder & Herder.

Gallagher, C. A. (1999). *Rethinking the color line: Readings in race and ethnicity*. Mountain View, CA: Mayfield Publishing.

Gallo, A. (2016, February 16). A refresher on statistical significance. Retrieved May 20, 2020, from https://hbr.org/2016/02/a-refresher-on-statistical-significance

Galvani, A. P., Parpia, A. S., Foster, E. M., Singer, B. H., & Fitzpatrick, M. C. (2020). Improving the prognosis of health care in the USA. *The Lancet*, 395(10223), 524–533. doi:10.1016/s0140-6736(doi:19)33019-3

Glaser, B. G., & Strauss, A. (1967). *The discovery of grounded theory: Strategies for qualitative research*. New York: Aldine Publishing.

Goffman, E. (1986). *Stigma: Notes on the management of spoiled identity*. New York: Touchstone.

Hazen, R. M. (2005). *Genesis: The scientific quest for life's origin*. Washington, DC: Joseph Henry Press.

Heller, D. (2000). *Speaking the unspeakable: An expensive truth–An exploration into the dynamics of sadistic and non-sadistic sexual and physical violence*. Paper presented to Danish Psychologists Union Meeting, Copenhagen, May 4, 2000.

Hinshaw, S. (2019). *Another kind of madness: A journey through the stigma and hope of mental illness*. New York: St. Martin's Griffin.

History of Science Society. (n.d.). An introduction to the history of science in non-western traditions. Retrieved May 18, 2020, from https://hssonline.org/resources/teaching/teaching_nonwestern/

Hochschild, A. R. (1990). *The second shift: Working parents and the revolution*. New York: Avon Books.

Hochschild, A. R. (2012a). *The managed heart: Commercialization of human feeling*. Berkeley, CA: University of California Press.

Hochschild, A. R. (2012b). *The outsourced self: Intimate life in market times*. New York: Metropolitan Books.

Hochschild, A. R. (2018). *Strangers in their own land: Anger and mourning on the American right*. New York: The New Press.

hooks, b. (1994). *Teaching to transgress: Education as the practice of freedom*. New York: Routledge.

hooks, b. (2003). *Teaching community. A pedagogy of hope*. New York: Routledge.

Horton, M., & Jacobs, D. (2003). *The Myles Horton reader: Education for social change*. Knoxville, TN: University of Tennessee Press.

Howard, R. (1981). One man scoops the experts. *In These Times*, March 31, 1981.

Hudson, B. (1975). Domains of evaluation. *Social Policy*, 6(2), 79–89.

Jacoby, R. (1985). *Social amnesia: A critique of conformist psychology from Adler to Lang*. Boston, MA: Beacon Press.

Jeffries, S. (2017, December 30). Psychopolitics: Neoliberalism and new technologies of power by Byung-Chul Han – review. Retrieved May 20, 2020, from https://www.theguardian.com/books/2017/dec/30/psychopolitics-neolberalism-new-technologies-byung-chul-han-review

Kelly-Irving, M., & Delpierre, C. (2019) A critique of the adverse childhood experiences framework in epidemiology and public health: Uses and misuses. *Social Policy and Society*. Retrieved from https://www.cambridge.org/core/journals/social-policy-and-society/article/critique-of-the-adverse-childhood-experiences-framework-in-epidemiology-and-public-health-uses-and-misuses/9D5EFAD918AAA52. Cambridge University Press. doi:10.1017/S1474746419000101

Khan Academy. (n.d.). *P-values and significance tests* (video). Retrieved May 20, 2020, from https://www.khanacademy.org/math/ap-statistics/tests-significance-ap/idea-significance-tests/v/p-values-and-significance-tests

Klein, N. (2014). *The shock doctrine: The rise of disaster capitalism.* London: Penguin.

Klein, N. (2020, May 08). Under cover of mass death, Andrew Cuomo calls in the billionaires to build a high-tech dystopia. Retrieved May 18, 2020, from https://theintercept.com/2020/05/08/andrew-cuomo-eric-schmidt-coronavirus-tech-shock-doctrine/?utm_medium=email&utm_source=The%2BIntercept%2BNewsletter

Kuhn, T. S. (1970). *The structure of scientific revolutions.* Chicago: University of Chicago Press.

Liebow, E. (1967). *Tally's corner a study of Negro street corner men.* Boston, MA: Little, Brown & Co.

Lipsitz, G. (2011). *How racism takes place.* Philadelphia, PA: Temple University Press.

Loevinger, J. (1976). *Ego development: Conceptions and themes.* San Francisco, CA: Jossey-Bass.

Lorde, A. (2017). *Your silence will not protect you.* London: Silver Press.

Mills, C. W. (1961). *The sociological imagination.* New York: Grove Press.

Nadel, L., Haims, J., & Stempson, R. (1992). *Sixth sense.* New York: Avon Books.

Nichols, J. (2018, August 2). Thanks to the Koch brothers, we have more proof that single payer saves money and cares for all of us. Retrieved May 18, 2020, from https://www.thenation.com/article/archive/thanks-koch-brothers-proof-single-payer-saves-money/

Nigam, V. (2018, December 4). Statistical tests - when to use which? Retrieved May 20, 2020, from https://towardsdatascience.com/statistical-tests-when-to-use-which-704557554740

P-values and significance tests (video). (n.d.). Retrieved from https://www.khanacademy.org/math/ap-statistics/tests-significance-ap/idea-significance-tests/v/p-values-and-significance-tests

Peterson, R. E., & Bilorusky, J. A. (1971). *May 1970: The campus aftermath of Cambodia and Kent State: A technical report.* Berkeley, CA: Carnegie Commission on Higher Education.

Polanyi, M. (1966). *The tacit dimension.* Garden City, N.Y: Doubleday.

Reich, R. (2018) The truth about privatization. Retrieved May 20, 2020, from https://www.nationofchange.org/2018/12/13/the-truth-about-privatization/

Rollins, J. (1985). *Between women: Domestics and their employers.* Philadelphia, PA: Temple University Press.

Schlipp, P. A. (1959). *Albert Einstein philosopher-scientist* (Vol. 1). New York: Harper.

Shabani, K. (2010). Vygotsky's zone of proximal development: Instructional implications and teachers' professional development. Retrieved from https://files.eric.ed.gov/fulltext/EJ1081990.pdf

Taylor, T. (1970, January 1). Robert Kennedy on shortcomings of GDP in 1968. Retrieved May 20, 2020, from http://conversableeconomist.blogspot.com/2012/01/robert-kennedy-on-shortcomings-of-gdp.html

Tse-Tung, M. (1966). *On practice.* New York: International Publishers.

Veysey, L. R. (1992). *The emergence of the American university.* Chicago: University of Chicago Press.

Vygotsky, L. (1978). *Mind in society: The development of higher psychological processes.* Cambridge, MA: Harvard University Press.

White, R. W. (1959). Motivation reconsidered: The concept of competence. *Psychological Review, 66*(5), 297–333. doi:10.1037/h0040934

Wolff, R. P., Moore, B., & Marcuse, H. (1969). *A critique of pure tolerance.* London: J. Cape.

Zuckerman, H. (1967). Nobel laureates in science: Patters of productivity, collaboration and authorship. Retrieved from https://www.jstor.org/stable/2091086?seq=1#page_scan_tab_contents

INDEX

activist 9, 11–14, 17, 26, 56, 130, 184;
   activism 3, 35, 211
African American 7, 32, 61, 89, 186, 194–5.
   Black 184, 191, 194–5
anomalies 23–5, 30. *see also* exceptions to
   the rule

Becker, H. 27, 29, 95, 109, 112
bias, biases, biased 18–20, 22, 28–9, 45–6,
   50–1, 56–7, 62, 82, 89, 93, 100, 106–7,
   112, 117–8, 132, 134, 144, 159, 171–2,
   201, 204, 206–7
bigger picture 8, 13, 20, 40, 46, 86, 108,
   175–6, 179–185, 198, 207, 210
both/and 115, 175, 189, 209
Butler, H. 6, 34–9, 127

collaborative 3, 11, 17, 20, 35, 65, 129, 133,
   146, 194, 199, 210
community agency 12, 56, 69, 101, 190; *see
   also* community organization, nonprofit.
community organization 54, 57, 68, 90,
   121, 134, 182, 199; *see also* community
   agency, nonprofit.
community services 34, 126; *see also* social
   services.
cost-benefit 160–1, 172, 202–3, 210
coronavirus 61, 175; *see also* COVID.
counseling 10, 35–6, 92, 94, 200; *see also*
   therapy, therapist.
COVID 2, 167, 211; *see also* coronavirus.
culture 27–8, 33, 37, 46–7, 52, 59, 60, 62,
   99, 132, 184, 191, 196, 207, 211

data analysis 79, 82, 84, 89, 104, 105,
   109–10
data collection 14, 64, 201; *see also* data
   gathering
data-gathering 18, 31, 63, 72, 79, 82–84,
   86, 103, 105, 110, 120, 162, 195, 208;
   see also data collection
democracy, democratic 9, 17, 34, 130, 176,
   185–6, 188, 206, 210
Dewey, J. 17, 22, 33–4, 43, 130, 196
disparities 61, 194–5
diversity 8, 9, 20, 73, 83, 103–4, 154, 171
Dreyfus, H., Dreyfus, S., Dreyfus model 22,
   36–9, 43–6, 110, 141–2

elders 65, 141, 204
emotion, emotions, emotional, emotionally
   2, 14, 22, 24, 37, 43–6, 75, 96, 145, 148,
   173, 189, 199, 200, 207
Ethics, ethical, ethically 2, 17, 20, 26,
   37, 87–8, 90, 99, 161, 176–7,
   198–203, 210
exceptions to the rule 8, 23–7, 30–1, 40, 78,
   83, 112, 143, 206
experimenting community 3, 35, 37–9
exploring, exploration 29, 31, 84–7, 89,
   116, 125, 126, 131, 180, 204

Freire, P. 17, 22, 33–4, 43, 47, 130

gender 9, 20, 46–7, 89, 154, 184, 186
government 2, 50, 54, 129, 136–7, 185
grounded theory 3, 13, 29, 41, 43, 82

history 3, 23, 26, 46, 58–62, 86–7, 107, 109, 135, 141, 196
Hochschild, A. 5, 27–8
homeless, homelessness 176, 182-3
housing 60, 65–6, 141
hypothesis, hypotheses 16, 27–9, 66, 88, 93–4, 112–3, 116–8, 134, 139, 151, 206

improvisation, improvisational 3, 8, 22, 33–5, 37–9, 41, 72, 96, 195, 206, 210
inclusive, inclusiveness 6, 8–11, 20, 48, 104, 145, 183, 185–6; *see also* multicultural.
inequality 18, 175, 183, 185
inspection 28, 111
interviewing 8, 12, 27, 72–3, 83, 89–90, 92–97, 99–102, 134, 142, 154

knowledge-building 12–13, 33, 129, 146–7, 176–7, 190, 192–3, 194–7, 206, 210
Kuhn, T. S. 22–26, 39, 43, 45–6, 52, 67, 107, 118

Loevinger, J. 22, 36–9, 43–4, 47

marginalized, marginalization 9, 11, 18, 20, 32–3, 46–8, 61–2, 146, 183–4, 185–6, 199–200, 202, 207, 211
multicultural, multiculturalism 6, 10–11, 48, 145, 183, 185–6; *see also* inclusive.

needs assessment 19, 132, 211
neoliberalism, neoliberal 175, 183, 185–6
nonprofit 10, 34, 181
note-taking 73, 78, 90, 98, 101–2

objective, objectivity 25, 34, 38, 58, 80, 106–7, 109–10, 139, 140, 144, 149, 159–160, 195, 203
own voice—*see* voice.

participant observation 12, 27, 72, 87–9, 109
participatory 10, 12–14, 17–8, 20, 90, 176, 182, 193–5, 198–9, 206, 211
privilege, privileged 7, 9, 20, 46–7, 50, 62, 185, 200, 202–3, 207

questioning 75, 88, 132, 143, 182; question-asking 67–8, 71; asking questions 8, 63, 65–9, 71, 104, 118, 128, 196, 204, 208

racism 31, 60, 183–4, 190–1
reliability 79–80, 104–7, 123–5, 139, 196

risk, risks 2, 61, 69, 88, 93, 103, 114. 137, 160–61, 172–3, 184, 199–201, 203, 208, 210

sampling, sample 8, 43, 64, 72–3, 81–6, 90, 104, 119, 125,144, 154–6, 165–6, 171, 208
sensitizing concept 29–32, 80–1, 86, 141, 191–2, 194, 205
social change 6, 9–11, 17, 23, 33, 57–8, 129–30, 138, 146, 150, 183; *see also* systemic
social justice 10–11, 17–18, 20, 59, 177, 186, 210
social responsibility 201–2, 204
social services 84, 183; *see also* community services.
somatic 11, 42–3
symbolic Interactionism 14, 27
systemic 46, 115, 182–3, 186, 192; *see also* social change.
statistics 64, 87, 109, 152–3, 159, 161, 170, 173, 207–8
stories 3, 8, 20, 23, 29, 31, 41, 45, 59, 123, 129, 132, 139–42, 144, 173, 177, 194, 195, 203, 206–7, 209–10; storytelling 139–40, 143, 194, 209

transparent, transparency 23, 29, 33, 105–6, 108–9, 117, 119, 128–9, 138, 140, 143, 145, 162, 199, 202–3, 206–209
teach, teachers, teaching 6–7. 9–10, 12, 19, 33–5, 47, 60–1, 77, 91, 94, 99–100, 118, 126–7, 138, 142, 145, 147, 183, 186–7, 193, 206, 211
therapy, therapist 10–11, 42–3, 92, 142; *see also* counseling.
think tank 129, 211

validity 13, 33, 74, 79–80, 104–9, 113, 115, 123–5, 127, 155, 170, 172, 193, 196, 201, 207, 209–10
violence 152, 166, 190, 209
voice (own voice) 5, 9, 12, 18, 21, 57, 94, 95, 140, 144–8, 177, 197
Vygotsky, L. 22, 36, 41–2, 44

Western Institute for Social Research, WISR 3, 5–7, 10–17, 30, 48, 65–6, 142, 145–7, 150, 176, 193–6, 204, 211

youth 26, 30, 60, 77, 203, 211

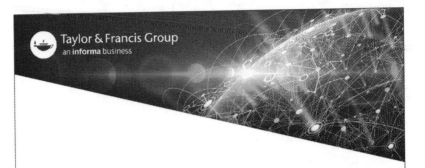

Printed in the United States
By Bookmasters